"*Behind the Curtain: A Peek at Life from within the ER* grabs you from the first page with its mix of all-too-real experiences and important life lessons from Dr. Jeffrey Sterling. With straightforward, pragmatic advice—"Stop smoking. Now."—and stories of the heroic efforts in hospital emergency rooms to save lives, Dr. Sterling gives the reader an inside look at the challenges and joys of life as an emergency room physician. His gentle wisdom, learned through years of extraordinarily difficult experiences, provides guidance for all who read this wonderful book."

—Morton Schapiro, PhD
President and professor
Northwestern University

"*Behind the Curtain* is one of those rare books that takes the reader into a fast-paced, unfamiliar setting through the eyes of the expert. Jeff has done an outstanding job of writing about his many years in ERs across the country. He also balances his life stories with a healthy dose of recommendations on how readers can easily avoid placing themselves in those dangerous and traumatic situations that often lead them to the ER and physicians who have to make the same split-second choices that Jeff has made for years to save lives."

—Harry Lennix
Veteran actor, director, and producer

"Behind the Curtain: A Peek at Life from within the ER is a riveting primer of the types of cases that place patients in the emergency room, but it goes much further in explaining how physicians operate in such unknown conditions to the betterment of their patients. Practicing medicine when you never know who will walk through the door or be brought in by ambulance is a constant, changing environment requiring split-second decisions. That's the fascinating expertise Dr. Sterling brings to the reader in recognizing the medical attention needed in the fast-paced world of the unknown that is the American emergency room."

—Rahn Kennedy Bailey, MD, DFAPA
113th President of the National Medical Association
Chairman of Psychiatry, Wake Forest Baptist Medical Center

"Authentic. This is how I would describe Jeff Sterling. Having known Jeff since the early days of his career, I immediately saw him as a leader who was knowledgeable and perceptive beyond his years. *Behind the Curtain* reads in the same manner in which Jeff speaks—straightforward. Dr. Sterling expresses high intelligence and demonstrates his observational skills about the people and situations with which he is confronted. This collection is infused with keen insights, singular observations, genuine compassion, and not-so-cryptic humor grown out of a rich array of personal pursuits and professional experiences. Still a leader, he continually aims to teach and to serve."

—Annette McLane
Associate Director for Programs and Conference Services
Student National Medical Association

BEHIND THE
CURTAIN

BEHIND THE CURTAIN

A Peek at Life from within the

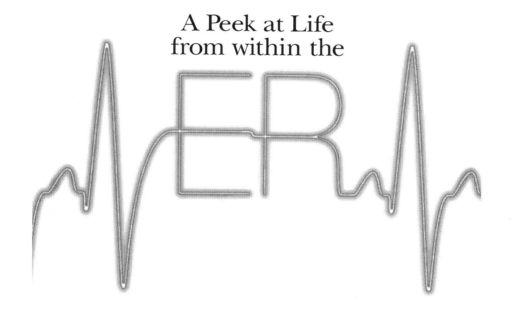

Jeffrey E. Sterling, MD, MPH

Behind the Curtain: A Peek at Life from within the ER

Brown Books Publishing Group
16250 Knoll Trail Drive, Suite 205
Dallas, Texas 75248
www.BrownBooks.com
(972) 381-0009
A New Era in Publishing™

ISBN 978-1541121485
LCCN 2015939716

Printed in the United States
10 9 8 7 6 5 4 3 2 1

For more information or to contact the author, please go to
www.JeffreySterlingBooks.com
www.JeffreySterlingMD.com

*I dedicate this to my wife, whose support
has allowed me to become everything I am.*

*I dedicate this to my mother and children
who keep me honoring the past and
looking forward to the future.*

Table of Contents

Acknowledgments

I offer special thanks to every patient that has allowed me to provide care and practice medicine. Although the nature of treating disease can be dehumanizing, your diversity has kept me grounded and constantly fascinated by human nature. Special thanks also go to my friends, colleagues, and Brown Books for the enthusiasm with which this project has been embraced.

Introduction

I have spent over twenty years as an emergency physician. I trained at one of the finest facilities in the country, the legendary Cook County Hospital in Chicago. I have served as head of nearly a dozen different emergency rooms (ERs) in six different states in virtually every societal setting, and I have overseen over twenty different ERs in varying leadership capacities. If I haven't seen it all, it's only because new diseases are being created.

The activities within emergency departments are mirrors to the real world and can also be viewed as society's truth serum. I am so glad my college major was in psychology and not in something like biology or chemistry. I have spent so much time dealing with the nuances and particulars of human behavior that I should have an honorary doctorate in psychology.

What happens "behind the curtain" is real. Often it's not the parts of society that are presented publicly for consumption. In the ER, physicians walk into a room and immediately get exposed to things that one would otherwise get arrested for seeing (at least without permission) and things that most normal people would shriek in horror from seeing. People are so desirous of help that they reveal it all and talk so honestly that police could only dream of getting such willing cooperation during their interrogations. Now, that doesn't always happen upfront, but the skilled emergency physician can most always get the story. It's a nice by-product of physiology that even if and when the patient is not truthful, his or her physical signs and symptoms also tell a story that, if you're paying attention, either does or doesn't support what's being said.

The emergency department team has to guard against becoming cynical, detached, and dehumanized by it all. The constant onslaught of human pain, suffering, and misery is a bit much to handle. The cynical emergency physician forgets that "Mr. Jones" exists and refers to him as "the drunk in Room Five." Even if one isn't cynical, he or she must learn to balance some hard truths. Many people often show up in an ER as victims of the consequences of their own actions:

- We eat too much.
- We drink and abuse drugs too much.
- We have inappropriate, unsafe sex too much.
- We beat up on each other too much, both physically and mentally.
- We're reckless in our handling of automobiles, guns, and other machinery.
- Worst of all, we don't engage in health prevention and present to the ER—the most expensive portal of entry to the healthcare system—only when a medical emergency has befallen us.

Behind the Curtain is a set of memorable stories and experiences that are rough approximations and conglomerates of over seventy-five thousand patients I have seen over the years. I hope they not only entertain you but also provide a peek into the experiences of both patients and healthcare providers. Who knows? Maybe you're not alone in what you feel or what you've done! Thanks to all my wonderful nurses, patients, and colleagues for providing me a journey worth sharing.

The Drop-Top Shaved Top

I t's my job to treat, not to judge, but sometimes it's very difficult because the emergency physician understands that risks are not just risks but instances of occurrences. In other words, if you introduce certain risks into your life, certain bad things are going to happen eventually.

There are certain things about driving that just aren't up for debate anymore. Driving without a seat belt. Drinking, texting, and other distracted driving habits. Driving a motorcycle without a helmet. And then there's drag racing on streets.

I recall being young and very impressionable in medicine, spending time both in a coroner's office and in emergency departments. I remember the fear, shock, awe, wonderment, and excitement associated with every single patient I saw in those early years, as my role in their care and my ability to occasionally make a difference became apparent to me. I also remember the bewilderment and frustration, not only from my inability to save certain individuals, but also from my inability to save certain individuals from themselves.

I will never forget the day a certain patient came in deceased from a motor vehicle crash (they're not accidents). He had been drag racing another vehicle on a crowded street, and his car flipped 180 degrees, leaving it upside down. The problem in this case was the drop-top portion of the vehicle was down. This gentleman came in with approximately three inches shaved evenly from the top of his scalp. Needless to say, he was dead on arrival.

Looking back, given the speed of the car and the mechanism of injury, I'm sure he died from a broken neck. I'm surprised he wasn't decapitated.

Part of being an emergency physician is mastering the art of knowing when to act and when not to act. We are always being put upon to "Don't just stand there. Do something!" when, in fact, in many cases the correct mantra is "Don't just do something! Stand there." Sometimes our actions interfere with the body's own efforts to recover, and inaction will actually allow things to get better. In other instances, it's honestly cruel to further assault someone who is dead and gone.

The surprising part about these particular injuries and deaths is that we too rarely take advantage of the lessons that are there to be learned. We appropriately spend time mourning the loss of the deceased but hesitate to speak ill of any of the habits that caused the preventable and premature death. I would respectfully suggest that a more complete mourning of those who die this way would include an assessment of lessons learned from their lives and how those of us who remain stand to benefit from how they lived—and how they died.

Focusing on the Trauma, Not the Drama: A Stab Wound to the Eye

One of the most important skills of the emergency physician is the ability to stay out of the moment. It's critical to stay above the fray and focus on the academics of the case. Otherwise, it's way too easy for the drama of the emergency room to resemble something out of a bad TV reality show or horror movie. That said, some presentations challenge and defy our best efforts.

Working in the ER on a weekend is challenging. Working in the ER overnight is unpredictable. Working in the ER in the summer means trauma. When you put all three together, all bets are off.

I vividly remember the feeling and the shift. While working in a small community hospital, on hour sixteen of a twenty-four-hour shift, I nervously laid my head down in anticipation of possibly getting a brief reprieve from the Chinese water torture flow of patients and being rewarded with a brief nap. Then the call came, seemingly as soon as my head hit the pillow. "Trauma One . . . Trauma One." *OK, so this is routine, right?* Nope. The nurses are banging on my door. That never happens. Nurses are great at letting you know when something is really going on.

Up I jump, and I immediately hear screaming. ERs are always loud, but this was a level of panic. At this point, I'm running to the trauma room (which never happens) and I'm watching a man faced with a decision no one should ever have to make. He has a knife through the top of his eye. His ongoing decision was whether to leave it in or snatch it out.

This is where the academic has to come out of the emergency physician. I'm not watching a horror movie. The concern is not a knife in the eye. The potential concern is called a *perforated globe*, and that's what management of the patient needs to be reduced to. It's always about the life threat first, then the limb threat, then everything else. In the midst of all the noise and drama, I think . . .

All trauma is the same at the beginning. Don't focus on the drama. Treat the patient with trauma. This means I need to make sure nothing has occurred that's even more important than a potential knife to the eye. *OK . . . His airway is intact. Check. He's breathing OK. Check. His blood pressure is normal. Check.* That's right. Even if there's a knife hanging out of your eye, it might not be the most important thing happening to you.

The really beautiful thing about a well-run emergency department is the poetry in motion that occurs. It's truly controlled chaos, with multiple things occurring simultaneously. I have the staff getting the surgeon on the phone. Since this small hospital is not a trauma center, he needs to be transferred out. The staff is getting the patient's clothes off to facilitate my exam and treatment. I get to stay in the zone, focus, think, control the scene, and act when needed.

Great. His clothes are off, and everyone is calm and working. I have both eyes covered—his, not mine (covering the unaffected eye restricts movement in the affected eye, which is important)—and the patient has been given medicine to relax. When I got to examine him, fortunately, this was a single wound without additional injury.

It's very true that trauma patients are incredibly lucky unless they aren't. Once the patient was relaxed enough to examine, I discovered that he had ducked just enough for the knife to lodge immediately above the eye into the bone. However, because of the downward thrust of the hand, the possibility still existed that damage had occurred to the eye and its supporting apparatus. So he got stabilized, packaged, and shipped to the big city trauma center, where everything ended up just fine.

All in a night's work.

Cockroaches

How would you respond if you had a cockroach inside of you? I have seen the entire range of emotions, from fear and anger to sadness and sobbing. I have seen them in the mouth, nose, and vagina. However, they mostly seem to inhabit the ears. This really freaks people out because they're having visions of cockroaches scratching and clawing and eating their way into the brain.

It's always in the middle of the night when you're asleep. Perhaps food was left on the bed next to you. Perhaps you didn't wash up after becoming adventurous with food. That attracts them. Then you're lying down with your mouth open and the rest of you exposed, and then it happens. An itch becomes horror.

I can only imagine the ride to the emergency room. That seems like a long time to yell and scream, but it must happen, because it's sure going on when they hit the door. Now, the adults are usually screaming, but the kids are eerily quiet, even if they're quiet because they're terrified.

So they come in, and it all ends very quickly. You take a second to look in the ear to see if it's alive or dead and to see if there is any damage to the eardrum. One of various solutions is placed in the ear canal to kill the cockroach; it then gets extracted with special tools. The screaming begins once the patient sees what was inside them; you'd think they'd turn away. That's usually followed by them slapping their head as if something's still inside them, with a request to recheck. It all gets better after about ten minutes.

I would imagine the ride home is almost as bad as the ride to the emergency room. How do you go back to sleep after that?

GSW to the Face:
He Actually Wanted to
Blow His Brains Out

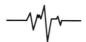

Nothing about an attempted suicide is a joke. That said, there are certain aspects of how people attempt to commit suicide that are surreal and defy logic. It seems that the subconscious battle between self-preservation and the desire to end one's life plays out in different ways. One example of this is the way some people attempt to "blow their brains out."

So here I am, a young physician, knowing just enough to both be dangerous and get lucky enough to save a life. During this phase of my existence, I spend a lot of time looking at the door. Why, you may ask? The specialty of emergency medicine is the acute management of whatever walks through the door. If you practice long enough and see enough patients, every conceivable presentation will walk through the door or be brought in by ambulance. In those early days, there were many nervous glances toward the door.

In a big-city trauma center, you seem to get either a little bit of notice about what's coming in or else panicked patients just running through the door. In this case, the call came in over the ambulance squawk box as, "Attempted Suicide, Gunshot Wound to the Face." That could mean a million different things:

The patient could be already dead.

The patient could be dead on arrival.

The patient could be brain dead.

The patient could be lucky—back to this in a moment.

In case you're wondering why more information isn't provided, it's because the paramedics are usually busy trying to save a life and aren't exactly free to chat.

The patient hits the door, and because it's a trauma, it doesn't matter if the patient put a bullet through his or her chest or stubbed a toe. We proceed according to the ABC's, which are A: an assessment of the **airway** (making sure there's no obstruction to the windpipe and checking the ability to speak), B: an assessment of **breathing** (making sure the lungs are OK), and C: an assessment of **circulation** (making sure there isn't a loss of heart function or blood that prevents oxygen and nutrients from getting around the body). Of course, while we're doing this, we are mindful that there's a gunshot wound somewhere. That fact can't distract us from the ABCs, injuries to which represent the final common pathways of death and must be stabilized first.

Now mind you, if you were watching this, your heart would be racing one hundred miles an hour. Everything is simultaneously chaotic and controlled. And then you would realize the manifestation of the subconscious battle that must occur in many patients who try to blow their brains out. They don't hold the gun to their forehead, temple, back of the head, or elsewhere where the brain may be located. They place the gun under their chin and tilt upwards. Of course, the action leans the head (and brain) back, away from where the gun is pointing. So now, "Attempted Suicide—Tried to Blow His Brains Out" becomes, "Attempted Suicide—Guy Blew His Chin and Mouth Off." The rest of the story involves efforts analogous to completing a jigsaw puzzle—looking for missing pieces and attempting to figure out what goes where and how sections connect. But hey, he's alive and did live to tell the story, although not for quite a while later.

8

Cracking Open a Chest

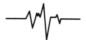

Some emergency rooms are not located in the safest communities. Metal detectors are increasingly common. Cars have famously crashed into hospital buildings. Stab wounds and gunshot wounds occur all around the hospital. So when you choose to work in such an environment, you kind of expect certain things to happen.

It's Friday night in the big city, which means anything is happening. It's just a matter of what will reach my emergency room. You can hear the screams from outside the door. "We need help. He's been shot!" *OK . . . that happens. We can deal with that. Sigh.* Still, patients don't realize the difference between regular hospitals and trauma centers. There are times when going to the closest facility is absolutely the right thing to do because the first order of business is to get stabilized. In other instances, you really need to be in a stroke center, a chest pain center, or a trauma center—not necessarily because of the physicians but because the resources these specialty hospitals are likely to offer are significantly different.

OK, so we have a gunshot wound, apparently to the chest. This is not good. No, actually it's catastrophic. The patient is out cold and doesn't have a pulse, whereas one existed right before coming into the emergency room.

Pause.

There are situations, particularly in the setting of trauma where the patient's only chance of life after death is a procedure called a *thoracotomy*. It is literally the opening up of the patient's chest wall to gain direct access to the heart, in order to repair it, relieve it of some obstruction, or directly stimulate it. There are a few instances in emergency medicine when we are permitted (actually expected) to do things that the first time you learn about them you'd think no human should be allowed to do to another person. Then you realize that you might actually snatch someone from the jaws of death if you just stay focused. That's when you've crossed over to the other side emotionally. Still, regardless of the need or ability to perform, cracking open someone's chest feels just like driving your car over a squirrel.

This happens so quickly that there's no time to do anything other than act. In order for the procedure to even have a chance to be successful, the patient basically has to have collapsed after experiencing very limited types of injuries almost immediately prior to arrival or upon arrival. It's a situation where the patient is dying and going to die without this effort being made. Even so, the success rate is close to 0 percent.

But still you proceed.

Everything is happening in slow motion, even while this is occurring in seconds:

- Intubate the patient (put the patient on a breathing machine).
- Clean and prepare the patient.
- Make the incision in the skin through the ribs, cutting the skin and through the muscles.
- Open the chest cavity (rib cage) and spread it open.
- *(Mental note: ignore all the sounds of ribs popping or breaking.)*
- Avoid the nerves and blood vessels.
- Evacuate any blood that obscures your view.
- Identify the heart and open the heart sac.
- Repair what you find and stimulate the heart.

It's rare that a trauma suite is quiet, especially during a resuscitation. However, those in the room can't help but be transfixed by the combination of the definitive nature of life and death in the balance, the preposterousness, shock, awe, and audacity to assault a human body this way, countered with the absolute necessity of giving the patient the best, last chance of survival.

I performed the procedure four times during my twenty years of practice. I never personally had a patient come back. I do know of two instances in which the procedure was successful. I'm not big on heroic efforts "when the time has come," but in the hands of an experienced emergency physician or trauma surgeon, I think I would want this done to me or my family. I also think I want to avoid being shot in the chest.

From the Jaws of Death

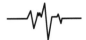

There's a line from the great movie *Groundhog Day* where Bill Murray's character muses, "Maybe God's not omnipotent. Maybe he's just been around so long he's seen everything." Part of the reality of cardiopulmonary resuscitation is there's data, and the emergency physician knows it. You understand the probability of survival based on several things: there's the time between the collapse and the arrival of the paramedics, the duration of time prior to arrival to the emergency room, and the types (and relative success) of efforts made in the field prior to arrival. Yet, even when it seems bleak, none of that deters you from always giving the patient the very best chance of survival once they arrive. As you might imagine, there's nothing as fulfilling for a physician as cheating death. When a patient is trying to die, it means a patient is going to die—unless you successfully intervene.

When that patient hits the door, I always look at the paramedics first. These guys are heroes, and they're our agents in the field. I have always spent a lot of time teaching and offering them tips so they can offer patients an even better chance of survival. They invariably will give me a look of "I have made you proud," "I need your help," or "There was nothing we could do." They're also either racing or strolling, which also tells me quite a bit.

I would bet emergency room resuscitations aren't what you think. Some of you know cardiopulmonary resuscitation (CPR). Some of you may even know advanced cardiac life support (ACLS). There's also Pediatric Advanced Life Support (PALS),

Advanced Trauma Life Support (ATLS), Neonatal Advanced Life Support (NALS), and others. This never-ending alphabet soup of protocols represents efforts to teach folks ranging from laymen to physicians how to handle life-threatening situations. Instead of just knowing those guidelines, your best emergency physicians understand the reasoning behind the guidelines; they know if and when to use them and when to deviate from them. I have had resuscitations last two minutes and others two hours based on the flow of a given case.

The important thing for me when beginning a resuscitation is to have already envisioned the process. I have hundreds of treatment algorithms racing in my head, and I'm prepared for a nearly unlimited set of eventualities. You never know for sure, but there are patients that you expect to save and bring back from death's door. I want to convey that optimism to my team. The room needs that positivity and everyone's best efforts. Additionally, I know I want this patient to either recover or die with dignity. I also know I want the family to understand what's happening as it is happening. Their input often provides valuable clues and can guide the length of the process if and when considerations such as medical futility come into play.

I think about the last patient I resuscitated. He hit the door with the paramedics racing in on the stretcher and pumping on his chest. They give me the look that says: "We didn't bring him back, but he's not dead." OK. *He's not going to die on my watch.* We get him in the room. The team is a well-oiled operation. There's plenty of noise in the room as every member performs his or her routine tasks. Someone's getting the IVs started. Two of them with big tubes for rapid fluid delivery. *Good.* Another nurse is getting information from the family that will be conveyed to me. *Good.* Another nurse is preparing the medicines and equipment she knows I will be using, and yet another is recording everything. My respiratory therapist is standing next to me, and the patient is being unclothed and connected to the monitors. That took about fifteen seconds. *This is beautiful.* All the noise stops when I speak. "Mr. Smith is going to make it out of here. Let's do this."

If it sounds in any way inappropriate to say such a thing, it's not. The team desperately wants to save every patient possible and needs to know I believe. My number-one rule in emergency medicine is "When it hits the fan, take your own pulse first." This has two meanings for me. If my pulse is still present, that means I'm going to be OK when this is over, so there's no reason for me to worry or not do the best I can. The additional meaning—that's applicable in this setting—is I need to remain calm. The staff is feeding off of me and looking to me for leadership. If I appear frazzled, and especially if it appears as if I don't know what I'm doing, things won't go well. That is a huge key to a successful resuscitation (and a successful emergency department as well).

We rapidly move to treatment. CPR is ongoing. A breathing tube is placed down the patient's throat to protect his airway from aspirating food from the adjacent *esophagus* (food pipe) as well as to keep him oxygenated. *No problems there, no problems exist with breathing.* We have two large-bore IVs in place. Although the heart monitor isn't showing a blood pressure, and we can't feel a pulse, there is a jagged rhythm on the screen that is consistent with *ventricular fibrillation* (or V-fib, as it's known). This is a heart rhythm in which the heart is basically quivering instead of delivering its normal strong, purposeful beats. These beats are needed to pump blood around the entire body, delivering the oxygen and nutrients the body needs to function. Ventricular fibrillation is ineffective and doesn't sufficiently contract the heart. It's unsustainable and will result in death if not converted back to a normal rhythm.

The paramedics chime back in. "Doc, he went in and out of this before we got here."

As I give the order to shock the heart (yes, we apply paddles and deliver energy to stimulate the heart), I take another good look at the patient. Although not young, he appears reasonably healthy. Any conscious efforts made by this non-obese, non-smoker to stay healthy despite whatever conditions led to this cardiac arrest are about to pay off in his having the best possible chance to make it through this.

It becomes necessary for me to place another access line in the patient, one that provides a more direct route to the heart (it's called a *central line* for that reason). This is necessary so the medicines that are about to be given can have a more rapid effect on the heart. It's a good thing this is done, because the V-fib didn't respond to the shocks as we had hoped.

The good news is, as soon as the line was in, we were able to give medicines that converted the V-fib to a normal heart rhythm, and this was accompanied by a return of his heart rate and a normal blood pressure.

All of this took about seven to ten minutes. The patient was taken to the Intensive Care Unit, and a nice long conversation was had with the family about what happened, his medical issues, and advance directives once this was all over with.

Meanwhile, back in the emergency department, no matter what else is going on, it is important to get the team back together, including the paramedics. These successes don't occur often enough, and when they do it is because of a team working together. Everyone needs their share of credit and praise, and the opportunity to ask questions and deliver teachable moments is best done in the wake of a success. It was a good day, and not just for the patient. I wonder what he's doing now.

Fighting Smokers for
Their Lives

As much as I love emergency medicine, I know I couldn't have gone into family medicine because of the smokers, if for no other reason. Anyone who knows me personally or professionally knows I constantly rant at smokers to save themselves. I simply know of no other thing we willingly do to ourselves to such devastating effect. By design, emergency medicine usually prevents physicians from developing the close relationship with patients that occur with primary care physicians. Yet even as an emergency physician, you still develop relationships with certain patients because they're always in the ER or because you had a particularly meaningful impact on their or their family's lives.

It has been close to being a joke with my various staffs over the years. I'm notorious for tying every possible malady to smoking. Had a dental abscess? Stop smoking. Bronchitis? Definitely stop smoking. Strep throat? How can you stand the taste? Asthma? You can't be serious. Pregnant? Do it for the baby. You're diabetic? Are you just asking for a heart attack? Even if you stubbed your toe, and I smell cigarette smoke. You do know that if no one smoked, one of every three cancers would not happen! Patients tiptoe around my emergency rooms, wondering if I'm working. They bring me progress reports and share their updates regarding their efforts to stop. On the other hand, I have been reminded many times that I'm not a primary care physician. But I am a public health professional, and smoking causes more annual deaths than HIV, illegal drug use, alcohol use, motor vehicle injuries, and gun-related injuries combined. So on I rant, because who exactly is being harmed by a physician telling them to stop killing themselves?

Aside from the public health considerations, I think fear may be in play here. Not for me, but from me for you. Seeing someone die while not being able to breathe, coughing up blood, and the rest that comes along with it has constantly been one of the most horrible experiences I have seen patients go through. I wouldn't wish that fate on anyone. Of course, when you're able to place a name and face to the circumstance, it's even worse.

In my experience, patients seem to do better quitting cold turkey, which is not to say that's the only way people succeed. It's just that quitting cold turkey occurs because someone is sufficiently motivated or forced, such as in the following examples:

- During pregnancy or after the birth of a first child.
- After a first heart attack or stroke.
- Once lung cancer, COPD, or another significant respiratory illness has developed.
- When they finally develop the will.
- Otherwise, when they die.

I had a wonderful relationship with an older lady who had been smoking for approximately fifty years. I had apparently done a good job with various family members, and she was the old-fashioned type that would bring pies (and later fruit!) to the emergency room. We had developed such a good relationship that she came to me one day and told me that because of me, she was going to give up cigarettes for New Year's, which was still a few months away. I had seen her often over the years but never for problems involving her lungs. I just remember she had an ongoing faint, soft cough and was frail. Because I could smell the cigarettes, that was enough for me to give her a pretty hard time about it whenever I saw her.

The next time I saw her, she had developed pneumonia. Since it was the first time I had seen her for a respiratory problem, it was the first time I had the opportunity to view a chest x-ray. Much to my chagrin, there appeared to be a lesion in her lungs that was suspicious for cancer. Hoping to disprove that, I ordered a CT scan, which has a higher level of accuracy in making this diagnosis. I really didn't need to see the result. I already knew. What made matters worse was knowing what the rest of her life was going to be. So many things we do in medicine, particularly emergency medicine, make us feel powerful and good about helping others. With cancer, that's rarely the case.

One other oddity about diagnosing cancer in the emergency department: many emergency physicians will not present you with the diagnosis, even if it is discovered. It brings such a level of emotion and so many questions that can't be immediately answered, it is generally thought best to leave such conversations to the primary care physician, who can spend time preparing and organizing the conversation and treatment strategy. Given that my patient was being admitted to the hospital, there wasn't going to be an inordinate delay in her receiving this information. Still, in this one instance in particular, I wish I had been able to share the diagnosis with my patient, simply because I was also in mourning about it.

Body Packers and Stuffers

You've probably heard the term "drug mule." I think the medical terms are even more interesting. These situations occur when someone is either prepared to take a trip (usually across a border) or is trying to escape the police.

You generally don't know that you're dealing with a drug mule until they're almost dead. Drug traffickers and their accomplices tend to play Russian roulette with information and keep it close to the vest until absolutely necessary. This can have deadly consequences. There are groups of symptoms that are associated with various drugs; they're called *toxidromes*. If you are familiar with the effects of various drugs, such as heroin or cocaine, you'd be close to understanding the effects of overdoses of these drugs. In an emergency room, in cases of overdoses that leave the patient in a coma, we are left to use these symptoms as clues to figure out what the patient took and how to treat him or her.

So I had this patient carried in to the emergency room looking like a character in *Alice in Wonderland*—mad as a hatter (displaying hyperactivity), dry as a bone (dry skin), red as a beet (flushed skin), blind as a bat (visual disturbances), and hot as hell (hot skin). You clue in pretty quickly on drugs like cocaine and methamphetamine, which stimulate the sympathetic nervous system and cause these symptoms.

At this point, job one is to get the patient under control both physically and physiologically. What this means is if the overdose is severe enough, the patient's vital signs such as heart rate and blood pressure can be dangerously high enough to create a life-threatening condition. It also means you can't effectively treat the patient until and unless you get this panicked, hyperactive patient under control.

After some sedatives and basic life-supportive measures do the trick of momentarily getting the patient under control, you try to figure out what's going on and determine if you're on the right track. There's no powder on this patient's nose. There's no evidence of fresh track marks (needle sticks). *Hmmm* . . .

Sometimes you have to impress upon friends and family that their loved one is about to die unless you can figure out what's going on. This message is typically offered more sternly based on the consequences of not knowing. Lying or withholding information from your emergency physician in the midst of a life-threatening condition is an incredibly dangerous and foolish decision. We're not the cops.

Drug traffickers come in many different varieties, but those who are drug mules are divided into "body packers" and "body stuffers." The body packer is the one who meticulously plans to smuggle. You'd expect the drugs to be securely double-wrapped and sealed before they're swallowed. Yep, they plan on retrieving them later, which is another reason why meticulous wrapping in multiple layers is necessary. I don't see these patients. Airport security or law enforcement catches them. I see the body stuffers.

The body stuffer is someone who is running from the police, trying to get rid of evidence, or a body packer who did a very poor job, allowing the contents to spill. If and when this occurs, it is the equivalent of a massive overdose and can be expected to become a medical emergency.

In an emergency room, it's a lot more likely that the unknown will kill you than even a massive overdose of a known substance. You just never know if there are multiple substances or an immediately deadly substance on board.

Once the "associates" finally let me in on what happened, the patient was appropriately treated, which resulted in a stay in the Intensive Care Unit along with a lot of handcuffs. But that's better than the alternative.

Handling Sexually
Transmitted Infections
in Young Men

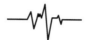

Psychologists will tell you that learning occurs better through positive reinforcement than negative reinforcement. I actually have a degree in psychology, so I know this to be true. However, that fact is not to say that negative reinforcement doesn't have its place.

The psychology of the young male is fascinating to see. It's not just that feelings of invincibility cause problems, but the decisions to act irresponsibly based on those feelings cause a lot of problems. When it comes to sexually transmitted infections (STIs), these actions can lead to lifelong impairment, and in the example of HIV/AIDS, even worse.

You should hear the conversations.

Hey, Doc. I think I caught something.

OK. What did you catch?

You know. I have some bumps down there.

Any discharge from your penis?

No. (He proudly holds back a smile.) But she does.

Have you had this before?

Sure, but I got it taken care of.

Do you wear condoms during sex?

Sometimes.

What does that mean—sometimes?

You know . . . When I think about it—but not with my girl.

How many sexual partners do you have?

(Generally three to six)

How many does she have?

Aww, Doc! What are you trying to say? It had better be one—just me!

Would you bet your life on it?

Ummm . . . nah . . . yeah! She's a good girl! But I wouldn't bet my life on anybody.

OK, because you are betting your life every time you have unprotected sex.

Aww, Doc! C'mon man. But I can get it treated . . . Right?

Once we get past the discussion that seems to go in one ear and out the other, the time comes to engage in diagnostic and treatment considerations. Because the discussion seems to go in one ear and out the other, often this will represent the best chance to reach patients. Treatment of STIs has gone through phases involving all needles, no needles, and considerations between those options. I have noticed over the course of my career that during the times when pills were used instead of needles, patients had much less of a deterrent, and I ended up seeing many of the same patients with regularity for subsequent STIs.

Medical reality has had a role in correcting how these patients are treated. STIs hang out like some type of gang. If you have one, you need to be treated for the rest, meaning the individual with any one STI is at a higher risk for having others. Practically, what this means is that it is a responsible course of action to test for and treat a wide range of STIs. This is good medicine as well as good public health; it is a high-yield activity to broadly treat individuals with risky behaviors.

Current treatment methods also appear to be a pretty good deterrent. Young males are not too fond of having multiple swabs inserted into their penises. It's not a well-kept secret among healthcare professionals that men are relatively more squeamish about taking injections than women. As drug-resistant strains of STIs have become more prominent and prevalent, injections have become more of a need.

Please don't read more into this than I intend. I don't believe many physicians are using injections and swabs as a deterrent to bad behavior. However, I do believe many patients seek to avoid these consequences of their bad behavior. I have had many patients tell me on subsequent visits for other reasons that they "saw me on their shoulder holding a needle" when they were making a decision to have sex (I think that was a compliment). If that works to save any patient from contracting HIV/AIDS, herpes, syphilis, gonorrhea, chlamydia, or any of the other sexually transmitted infections, then that's a good lesson learned.

When Big Is Not Fat

Families are fascinating when they accompany a loved one to the emergency room. In the effort to make sure nothing goes wrong, I see and hear everything from "Dr. Mom" to "This happened to my cousin once" to "I saw this on TV." And, of course, these days everyone is confronting you with whatever information they obtained from the Internet. These and many other ways of "helping" occur so much that the patient often can't tell his or her own story. This syndrome is even more prominent when there's someone in the family who works somewhere in the hospital.

I had a rather obese young lady in her twenties come in accompanied by her family. The family was somewhat anxious. She had been having abdominal pain for the last day, and it was becoming progressively worse.

- The mother wanted to tell me about how all the women in the family had gallstones.
- The sister wanted to tell me about her case of appendicitis.
- The patient thought she had a urinary tract infection (UTI) because she had been leaking urine.

The ironic thing about all of this is that families are often right, and as a physician, you ignore them at your own risk. The only time this really becomes a problem is when emergencies exist and inquiring minds get in the way of your efforts to assess the patient.

In this instance, the patient was obviously uncomfortable, but only intermittently. I was able to talk to her and the family for about a minute when she screamed. I interrupted the interview and started examining her belly.

Wow.

When was your last period?

I don't know. I never have periods. What's wrong?

I call my nurse, who clears the family out so I can complete a pelvic examination. Believe it or not, I barely have time to get anything else done when a baby's head starts protruding through the vagina.

This obese woman with would-be gallstones, appendicitis, or a UTI was presenting with a term pregnancy, ready to deliver, with the mother never having known she was pregnant. The unfortunate thing was that by not knowing she was pregnant, the mother placed the newborn at all kinds of risks. Over a nine-month period of time, not only was there no prenatal care, she hadn't engaged in any health care.

The good news was that she appeared to have a supportive, loving family, and we delivered a healthy baby that day. Of course, as the family left the emergency room and made their way toward the obstetrics ward, I thanked the various family members for their input. In the final analysis, their not knowing what was going on was completely irrelevant. They're not physicians and aren't supposed to know what I know. What was important was that they cared enough to get her the attention she needed. There are far too many instances in which that is not the case.

Real Sex to the Extreme?

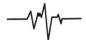

So I'm in a place that you think would be about as conservative of a place as exists in the US, true "rural America," as they say. It's Sunday morning, which in Texas is usually a slow time because most everyone's in church, headed to church, or getting ready for a Cowboys game.

Well, in comes a beautiful couple, straight out of central casting for "American family values." There's not much to think of until the conversation begins, although I should have been suspicious. Young men really represent the group least likely to utilize the ER, and when they do, it's usually for "man-type" activities. This gentleman wasn't bleeding, so who knew?

Anyway, they get straight to the point. During sexual experimentation in the middle of the night, after watching a provocative cable TV program, the wife slipped a raw potato in the husband's backside (intentionally and consensually, I might add). Given that it's not my job to judge but to treat, I do what we have to do. Removal of foreign bodies from the anus and rectum involves numbing and relaxing the nerves and muscles of the area, followed by insertion of an anal speculum (women will recognize the equivalent device used during gynecological exams) to open up the area for inspection and removal of the lodged foreign objects.

In these instances, people always wait a few hours to come to the ER as if the inserted object is going to come out on its own or will come out with the next bowel movement. Of course, it didn't, so back to the story. After inserting the anoscope and getting to work, I knew this wouldn't end well when the clamped tools I was using to remove the potato were bringing back only the equivalent of french fries. When this occurs, the next step is to send the patient up to the operating room, where more definitive medicine is given to relax the patient and extract what needs to come out.

Of course, I never saw the patient again, but I imagine he's doing well and the family is living happily ever after. I guess the lesson here is don't start something that you aren't prepared to finish, and don't get into a situation that you don't know how to get out of . . .

Epilogue. I would like to give a special thanks to the surgical team for the gift of a plate of baked potatoes they sent down to the ER for lunch!

Teens and Toes

This is a story about teens, which I'm sure conjures up a certain visual. It's also a story about how in an emergency department, doctors and patients are often concerned about different things altogether. Whereas physicians think about health, disease, and death, often patients are much more in tune with "quality-of-life" issues.

I remember a cute, stereotypically bubbly and exuberant young lady who came into the emergency department with her family during a very busy time, meaning she must have had to wait quite a while to be seen. I remember being impressed by her patience. Seeing her was actually a very pleasant interaction and a nice distraction from an otherwise busy day. I always like patients who manage to still have a smile on their faces or have pleasant personalities. As I'm greeting her, I'm imagining what her issue might be. Maybe she has a rash or a "female issue."

I ask her why she came to the emergency department; she plops her foot on the bed and takes off her shoes and socks. I'm expecting a splinter, especially painful corns, an ingrown toenail, or some other urgent podiatric concern. No. She has six toes, but nothing else appears to be immediately problematic that I can see.

OK. What can I do for you?

I want that extra toe off.

OK. Have you discussed this with your doctor?

Yes, but I want it off now! It's gross!

There's always someone screaming in a busy emergency department. Over time, you learn to phase out the noise and categorize different types of sounds so as to know which ones may require special or immediate attention. It's all about prioritization. Right about now, every other sound in the emergency department has just become magnified.

Yet, this young lady is presently in front of me. Her concern is legitimate to her and deserves a serious conversation. Yes, even though a young lady has tolerated a sixth toe for sixteen years, once she has decided it needs to be gone today, it becomes her emergency. Trying to explain to her that it is still a cosmetic concern and not a life-threatening emergency is a more difficult conversation than you might think. That doesn't mean anything is going to be done about it today, but her concerns still need to be respected.

Instead of confronting or even engaging her about the impossibility of her concern being addressed immediately, I let her know that I'm going to work for her to coordinate some things with her primary care physician. This immediately diffuses a potentially volatile situation—it could become volatile if she perceives I am rendering her and her concern unimportant, and it could become volatile if I succumb to the inclination to tell her this isn't an emergency and needs to be addressed elsewhere.

About 80 percent of the things for which people come to the emergency department aren't emergencies or even potentially life-threatening conditions. This means they could be addressed elsewhere. However, there's a huge convenience factor in using the emergency department. It's relatively quick and often more definitive in getting to the bottom of various issues than a single visit to your primary care doctor. This is completely consistent with the new prevailing culture of quick fixes and instant gratification. I think the terms emergency room and emergency department should be replaced by "acute care center" because that's actually what they have become. Hospitals are especially keen on retaining all the business they can because they're actually in business. It's bad business to turn any type of paying patients away. That's why customer satisfaction initiatives don't distinguish between those with "true emergencies" and those presenting for convenience concerns. It's all the same, and as long as hospitals are allowed to charge higher rates for the same concern to be seen in the hospital setting as opposed to the clinic setting, it will continue.

I spoke with the young lady's primary care doctor, who was aware of all of this and basically blew it all off, saying, "Things are in the works to address it." He knew why I had to call. Meanwhile, the young lady and her family were pleased that progress was being made toward getting the extra toe removed. She was an attractive young lady maturing into a beautiful woman, and her concern, even though it wasn't a medical emergency, was still a need to be addressed. Emergency rooms still assume part of the role in facilitating primary care.

However, as I left the room and reentered my loud and busy department, I couldn't help but think, *I wonder if any of them have any clue how much that just cost . . .*

Giving Birth to a Seizure

I think the phrase "the calm before the storm" was created in an emergency department. One day, as our staff sat down to chomp down lunch in the thirty seconds we had anticipated we might have before the next emergency, we were almost made to choke on our food.

An entire family barreled into the emergency room with a new mother; she had delivered her first child approximately eight hours ago. The family thought she was sleeping, but upon checking on the crying baby, they found the mother having a seizure. She did not have any history of seizures, and they said her pregnancy was unremarkable except for some concerns about high blood pressure. This family meant business and meant to be intimidating. They were yelling, "What did you do to her?" *Wait, we didn't deliver this woman's baby, but I know what they mean. This woman's life is in danger . . .*

Childbirth is usually a joyous time in a family's life, and one would think any anxiety associated with that timeframe would be related to adequate care of the newborn. Yet, there are instances in which the problems after delivery belong to the mother.

This presentation is a pretty good example of how emergency medicine works. We often don't have the luxury of time to get extensive histories on patients or order a battery of tests to help in making a diagnosis or beginning treatment. To do so in this circumstance would likely mean the death of a new mother. Instead, circumstances reflect probabilities and priorities. Conditions that are life-threatening and possible within a clinical scenario are the highest priority to treat immediately.

Emergency physicians also operate with hundreds of algorithms in their heads that are triggered by symptoms or word associations (a.k.a., "the sticker on the patient's forehead" or "the bizz-buzz," respectively). Despite the intensity and danger present, this case is reducible to *postpartum* (after delivery) *seizures*. In the world of emergency medicine, this means *eclampsia* until and unless proven otherwise. Nothing else matters. Not even if you had told me she has a history of seizures and hadn't been taking her medicine. The life threat comes first. Even if she had a giant nail sticking out of her foot at the same time.

Eclampsia is a complication of pregnancy-induced high blood pressure with the signature symptom of seizures usually in the second half of pregnancy or shortly after delivery. Because of the ability to prevent it during labor and delivery, most cases are now actually seen after delivery.

It is critical to get medicines on board to control the seizures and to manage the blood pressure if it's still high. If this had happened while she was still pregnant, delivery would have been the cure.

Her symptoms are managed, and she ends up doing fine. At this point, there's not much to do other than observe her. The time to have made a difference was early in the pregnancy. Eclampsia and the preceding condition, *preeclampsia*, are best controlled by early and ongoing prenatal care.

The family is still furious after it's all done on our end. They're railing about mistakes made during the delivery and lawsuits against the hospital and the obstetrician. The notion that their loved one's life has just been saved or that perhaps just one ounce of prevention could have prevented any of this never occurred to them. Knowingly and thankfully, there always seems to be at least one person in the family who sneaks away to say "thank you." That really does mean a lot to us.

On to the next group of patients.

It's Still My Family

I have cared for children of multiple age groups who were victims of various types of abuse. Have you ever talked to a child who has been the victim of physical, sexual, or emotional abuse? It's not at all what I would have expected going into the situation the first time.

We greatly underestimate the "blank slate" that children are. In a country of over three hundred million individuals, it is a mistake to presume that every family is raising children according to the same script or that we even share the same aspirations for our children. This means parents have vastly different approaches in raising or "handling" their children. There is no universal trigger that leads a child to become some homogenized version of an adult. We become what we learn to be. These considerations also play out in the values children acquire. As long as they receive some version of love, affection, food, and shelter from their parents, they can learn to interpret the circumstances of their lives as normal.

Overwhelmingly, children of abuse are discovered. It's not as if the kids realize something is wrong and complain to the authorities themselves, although physical abuse does have a greater chance of being caught. People make a big deal about how withdrawn children of abuse are. Some portion of that is because you are the stranger. Maybe you have just ripped them out of the only world they knew and they are being poked and evaluated as if they were aliens. Imagine how withdrawn you would be if you were airlifted and dropped off in New Guinea.

I recall an early evaluation of a seven-year-old child brought in by the Department of Children and Family Services. She was under protective custody because it had been discovered that she was getting spanked with some frequency, and it was deemed inappropriate. The evaluation included tag-team efforts by multiple professionals. Looking back, it had to be pretty intimidating because none of the family members were involved. The pediatric psychological counselor was asking questions in-between my doing the same while performing a physical examination.

I recall being stopped dead in my tracks during the conversation.

> Counselor: We're going to make sure no one hurts you, OK?

> Child: OK.

> Counselor: Sometimes bad people do bad things to children, and we can't let that happen.

> Child: Are you talking about my daddy?

> Counselor: Anybody that hurts you can't be allowed to do that.

> Child (in a hushed voice): It's still my family.

There are no easy answers to issues of abuse. We have made decisions as a society about when and how protective custody has a role. We must continue to be diligent to not exclusively focus on the child's physical well-being and not be mindful of their mental well-being. It would be prudent to have more conversations about the specifics of what is and isn't permissible in the raising and disciplining of children. These decisions need to be weighed based on the consequences of permanently displacing children from their families. Failure to do this with appropriate consideration can lead to a lifetime in which all that was accomplished was replacing one set of problems for another.

Finishing the Job

If you think about it, ERs (and particularly trauma centers) can be pretty dangerous places. Often the victims of trauma represent unfinished jobs, which is to say, in many instances someone intended for these patients to be dead. Every now and again, they come to the ER to finish the job.

I think back to the days before it was common to have metal detectors at the entrances of certain large ERs. I recall when ERs didn't have to be locked down as a routine. My mind wanders back to how patient intake would occur. When a patient registers to be seen and gets placed into an ER bed, that is when they're asked to disrobe and put on a gown. I always thought it to be an odd thing when, even after a patient was wearing only a gown, we would discover a machete or a gun still on their person. This actually happened to me on five or six different occasions! It's amazing how laissez-faire we were about such things. Maybe it was because those were the days when no one would ever think about hurting a doctor or a nurse. Curiously, in these instances, there were only two levels of concerns expressed by the patient. The first was some variety of "Doc, that doesn't get reported to the police, right?" The second was "You're gonna put that somewhere that I can get at it if I need it, right?" We always thought that second question was a joke—until it wasn't.

I recall a rather nondescript day in a large ER (in the staff's opinion, although the lay person would still be shocked at what was going on). We had numerous trauma patients being cared for, including one from whom we had confiscated a weapon. Our visitation policies were shockingly permissive; after all, these were "victims of trauma," and receiving social support during these times was thought to be the thing to do. Imagine how you would feel if your loved one was shot and you weren't allowed back to see him or her immediately. We thought we were helping by allowing visitors back so readily.

As was usually the case, "friends and family" were let back to see this patient; almost instantly you could hear yelling, screaming, and items being knocked to the ground, as if the patient were being assaulted with a knife.

This is where things get interesting in an ER. There are multiple considerations that must be addressed that constitute "the correct response."

- The staff is rarely if ever going to intervene in these situations in a way that places them in harm's way. Either your ER has a security force that can intervene in a timely manner, or you're likely out of luck unless you can adequately stave off the attack.
- The staff is obviously concerned with the patient. If something can be done for the patient without placing one's self at risk, it will be, although given the circumstances, it occurs less than you might think. Hospitals invariably have an emergency code designation that will be activated under these circumstances, but given the swift action of deadly violence, these efforts will most likely result in containment rather than prevention.
- The staff also is very concerned with the well-being of the other patients and their visitors. In fact, efforts to contain the violence and damage will often seem as important as addressing the situation at hand.

Fortunately, at this hospital a rather robust security presence was in effect, so the patient (who came to the ER after an initial stab wound) got away with only a second stab wound to the thigh and some other bruises. Needless to say, the staff was emotionally devastated by the episode. Even so, that memory serves in stark contrast to the day when a nurse was murdered literally in the office directly below me while I was in my office working. That episode made national news, including the front page of several prominent newspapers.

The ER is a place where the employees are constantly at risk. Patients and their families are concerned, fearful, and afraid for their well-being, but so is the ER staff. We have to deal with the burden of continual exposure to infectious disease, needle sticks, and physical harm. It shouldn't come as a surprise that ER staffs figure prominently in data when it comes to those at higher risk for suicide, drug use, depression, and divorce. In fact, it sounds a lot like a brand of post-traumatic stress disorder.

Next time you're in the ER, give your nurse, doctor, and other staff members a pat on the back and a "thank you." It will be more appreciated than you probably imagine. If you're a patient or a family member, work with us; we just want to be effective at a tough job.

Diabetic Feet

Not everything that comes to the emergency room is an emergency, although many of these things will end up as such if you let them linger long enough. In fact, about 80 percent of presentations could and maybe should be handled in a setting like a primary care office. A more important consideration is that many patients use the emergency department because of the absolute or relative unavailability of primary care physicians. This reality has consequences for patients with manageable diseases such as high blood pressure or diabetes.

In a word, diabetes is insidious. The disease just continues to progress with time, especially if you either don't control your diet and weight or if you're not compliant with your medication. I often wonder why certain diabetics don't just give up hope. I recall a patient I would frequently see in the emergency room whom I would warn and advise and with whom I would discuss how to avoid skin infections and foot ulcers because they lead to those all-too-frequent foot and leg amputations. He was pretty laissez-faire about it all and had horrible control of his blood glucose levels. Then came the last day I saw him. I knew what was going to happen shortly into our visit.

He found himself increasingly unable to walk due to pain in his left leg over the last "couple of weeks" and was starting to feel sick. He couldn't tell me much else. Emergency medicine is interesting in many ways; one of them is the need to rule out life-threatening conditions before routine, common, and maybe even obvious causes of illness. I had a few dozen questions that I wanted to ask, but knowing him, it was easier to start by looking him over while talking.

This could have been one of many things. I was hoping that it was a condition as simple as a disruption in the nerves of the legs, called *diabetic neuropathy*. This occurs in most diabetics over time and is accelerated in those who don't adequately care for themselves. That's an example of the routine and common explanation. *I will deal with that as a consideration later.* My real fear is he's done something that's life- or limb-threatening. Because diabetics have a loss of sensation in their feet, he may be unaware of an injury.

Although his pain is scattered across his leg, my eyes are drawn to his feet like a moth to a flame. The bizz-buzz of diabetics and leg pain is the diabetic foot ulcer. If you miss it, and even when you don't, there's a risk of a simple sore, scratch, or bump becoming infected and developing into an ulcer. Subsequently, the infection can go unrecognized and expand out of control, involving the bone and eventually leading to an amputated foot and/or other portions of the leg. As he unclothed and I took off his musty sock, my eyes tracked down his leg. I saw the redness and dried pus on the sock, leading to violent-appearing redness and more pus on the foot, all leading to a hole in the weight-bearing portion of his foot. Without thinking, I blurted out, "Did you even look at this?"

Given that I had seen him several times before, I knew that I had told him what I tell every diabetic I see in the emergency room. "Check your feet every day of your life, and have someone else look at them if you can't. Wear shoes when you're walking. Touch the water of your bath with your hands before you place your feet in."

He obviously wasn't doing any of this.

His examination revealed he had a fever. To make matters worse, he also had about a two-inch splinter in his foot. He had no idea it was there or any recollection of hurting his foot. His tests suggested he had a bone infection. *This isn't good.* Advanced diabetics are slow healers because of poor circulation to the distant parts of their bodies. Smoking makes this worse.

As I explained everything to him, I felt like I was talking to a wall or a man thinking about what he wanted for his last meal. *I know he's not tuning me out. He's just tuned out. It's as if he already knew and was afraid to find out.* That's why people "hate doctors" and "hate going to the hospital because that's where all the diseases are." No. Actually, you already have the disease, and you bring it to the hospital to get discovered before you die from it. After I finished talking to him, he looked up at me.

What do you think his first question was?

"Doc, can I go outside and smoke a cigarette?"

Pumping Someone's Stomach

—♒︎—

Timeline: Late Saturday night
Location: Any city, USA

The ambulance comes roaring into the hospital, bringing in an approximately twenty-year-old female who allegedly attempted suicide by the ingestion of a large quantity of unknown pills. Her life hangs in the balance.

The emergency department staff stands ready to act, armed to restrain her, pump her stomach, and pour activated charcoal down her Ewald tube.

Wait . . . this just coming in . . . we don't do that anymore.

Huh?

One of the things I never liked much about practicing medicine is when what is acknowledged as medical gospel sometimes becomes instantly extinct. The preponderance of evidence against an established course of treatment rarely shifts overnight, but if a landmark medical study suggests an abrupt change of course is in order, it will happen. Of course, that makes you concerned about how much we actually know; the actions we take (particularly in emergencies) need to be done so decisively and with such conviction that certainty about the existing medical literature is vital to those of us asked to do things for and to patients.

Still, it is simply amazing that in my career as a physician, the pendulum seems to have swung in many cases from "Don't just stand there. Do something!" to "Don't just do something. Stand there!" There are many examples of prior treatments that not only aren't done anymore but are now considered potentially dangerous. Patients with certain injuries that used to mean automatic surgeries are now observed. Broken bones and damaged ligaments are sent home for follow-up several days down the road. Infections that used to be treated in the Intensive Care Unit are now treated on the medical floor; infections that used to be treated on the medical floors are now sent home with oral antibiotics.

Another prominent example of this was the use of the *Ewald tube*. Most of you have probably never heard of it. Many of you have had a *nasogastric tube*—you know, those little rubber tubes that get run down your nose and throat into your stomach—if you had bleeding from your stomach or other conditions like pancreatitis or a small bowel obstruction. Well, an Ewald tube is a big rubber tube, about three times the size of a nasogastric tube, that you'd have to swallow. If you couldn't swallow it, we would put it down for you. The purpose of passing an Ewald tube down you would be to suck out pills and pill fragments if you had attempted suicide by swallowing a lot of pills. This used to be known as "pumping your stomach."

Receiving and placing an Ewald tube was a horrible experience. It felt like we were assaulting the patient. I used to wonder if its use was primarily as a behavioral deterrent (i.e., punishment) for daring to swallow all of those pills. In instances in which those attempting suicide did so to attract attention, this procedure certainly accomplished that particular goal.

Seemingly all at once, the powers that be in the world of toxicology decided that the body of evidence no longer warranted the use of Ewald tubes or pumping the stomach unless it was an imminently life-threatening circumstance. So, what exactly was the situation before? What about all those pills we were evacuating?

Today, the patient receives an antidote if one exists for the ingestion, supportive care for the effects of the ingestion, and in many cases he or she is allowed to drink the liquid charcoal preparation, which absorbs many different types of medicines and rapidly passes them through the system. Funny thing. There's not much difference in patient outcomes from the old days.

Devoured from Within

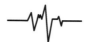

Medicine has affected me in some subtle yet unique ways. I have learned the range of human capability, both in positive and negative ways. I don't think it has made me cynical at all. What it has done is make me aware. However, I had to get to that point. As a young physician, there were many steps I had to take to realize that I wasn't part of an ongoing freak show, but I actually was front row, center seat to what and how life really is. I'm not the one trapped in *The Matrix*.

Medicine has also altered how I breathe. Smells are important in emergency medicine. They provide clues to disease. For example, cyanide smells like bitter almonds, and especially sick diabetics can have a musty, fruity smell on their breath. I notice I intermittently switch my breathing pattern to use short, rapid breaths in order to avoid certain smells. That is a mandatory skill in the emergency department, where poopy diapers, unkempt adults, bloody victims of trauma, toxic spills, and vomiting alcoholics present. There's just one thing about these types of patients, though. They can all be cleaned up. There are other smells that can't be cleaned or covered up.

One day, I walked out of one patient's room into the main ER area, and I was stopped dead in my tracks by a completely unfamiliar smell. By the time the nurse told me the patient was ready for me, I had already grabbed a mask, but the smell was still there. It was that kind of smell that makes you dizzy. I'm thinking, *This can't have been new. Why did it take so long for them to get her over here to be seen? And why wasn't she cleaned first?*

One thing the really old and the really young have in common is that when they are really ill, they have a limited set of responses. The elderly often just become listless. This isn't a good thing because what is needed is to yell and scream for attention; otherwise, in the worst of circumstances, they can be left in this condition until and unless discovered by someone else.

There was no history available from the nursing home other than "lethargic with AMS (altered mental status)," which could mean a hundred different things, so this is when the emergency physician has to go into detective mode. A large percentage of these patients in this age group end up with urinary tract infections, so I'm prepared for that possibility. I think I smell urine and feces, but some of that always seems to be there.

Another thing the elderly and infants have in common is that bad things often happen under the diaper. Remember that the next time you bring either to the emergency room, because if the patient isn't undressed, something could end up being missed. Noticing there's still a diaper on, I have the nurse help reposition the patient so I can get it off and complete the exam. I notice a bedsore.

Bedsores are very bad news. Bedsores positioned on the buttocks are a tragedy waiting to happen. They take on a life of their own. Because they are located on a weight-bearing part of the body, it's hard to get relief from them. Because of the position near the anus and vagina (think stools and urine), the infection can continue, spread, and extend.

The sore gets examined, and I discover a cavity up into the sore. Within the cavity, I see maggots. There's really nothing else to see or say. I look at the patient, look at the nurse, and leave the room. I ask the nurse to get the patient cleaned, and I ask another nurse to get elder protective services on the phone. The human part of me wants to be furious, but in the moment, that accomplishes nothing. This patient needs help, and I'm the one charged with getting it done. It is obvious (and later confirmed) that this lady has no one who visits or cares for her beyond what the nursing home offers.

I wonder how hardened you must be to abandon your parents when they're elderly. I also wonder how incompetent you must be to be charged with caring for them and be neglectful.

The existence of both realities is a disgusting part of our reality that is addressed far too infrequently. By no means is this meant to suggest this is the routine course of interactions between families and elderly parents or nursing homes and patients. But the fact that it can and does occur means we must be diligent in enforcing fundamental patient protections in these populations.

The patient was admitted to the hospital, requiring surgical cleansing of the area, antibiotics, and a long stay. There are a lot of circumstances in medicine in which, after treatment, patients are returned to the conditions that produced the pathology in the first place. That can't be right. We can do better.

Why Were You Up There?

One of the frustrations physicians have with patients is that many too often think linearly when it comes to health issues. You think you can smoke because you know someone who was a smoker and lived to be ninety years old. You think you read something on the Internet that sounds like what you have; thus, it automatically must be what you have. You think that if you get hit in the left side of your jaw, the injury must be on the left side of your jaw. Sometimes these things happen, but often it's not the case.

I once saw a guy who jumped off a roof after being startled. He landed on his feet after about a twenty-foot fall. He was brought in by ambulance in obvious pain. The foremost concern of the family was whether or not he had broken his feet. Sure he did. They told me as soon as he came in that they didn't want any other tests done. In discussing the risks with the patient, he and I decided that additional tests were needed and appropriate. A few weeks later, the family was absolutely furious upon receiving the hospital bill. The particular concern was "all the other x-rays." He clearly landed on his feet and didn't have any other complaints. Why were these other tests needed?

This brings to mind an applicable rule of emergency medicine:

Your physical problems aren't necessarily our priorities.

That's an affirmative comment, not one meant to imply a disregard of your concerns. It's a reminder that the priority in an emergency department is always the life- or limb-threatening condition to the detriment of an obvious and even dramatic injury. In the example of the above patient, it would be a breach of the emergency medicine standard of care not to fully examine and obtain x-rays of the spinal cord in a patient who fell from more than twelve feet. Even when you don't land on your back, such injuries are not only priorities to exclude, they're actually common. When you land on your feet, you transmit energy straight up your spinal cord into your back, which can result in fractures. Now imagine a fracture in your back that damages one of the nerves of your spinal cord. Now imagine partial or total paralysis that resulted from the injury. Now imagine that your emergency physician didn't order those x-rays. That's called medical malpractice, regardless of what the family told you to do (unless they held medical power of attorney over the patient, which wasn't the case here).

In the final analysis, the patient and the physician have the relationship, not the patient and the family. I can recall many cases in which the patient told me the true story or asked to have something done only once the rest of the family was out of the room.

Regarding the question "Why were you up there?," you never would have guessed that the patient was on the roof because it was his escape from the rest of the family. He even hid a cooler up there! Is a "Man Roof" a thing?

Now That's Some Bull!

It's not my job to judge, but to treat. I actually have learned to enjoy the diversity of experience gained from working all over the country. Still, there are things that we should be able to look at on an absolute scale and say, "Why would anyone do that?"

- I have cared for thrill seekers in the North who chased tornados.
- I have cared for five-year-old children in the West who presented with injuries while learning gun safety.
- I have cared for folks in the East who swam naked in the ocean on New Year's Eve.

On another occasion in the South, I had a seventeen-year-old cowboy walk in. It all looked very normal until I realized he was bleeding. Well, there had been a major rodeo nearby. Apparently, this young man was a past champion bull rider, and his huge, gorgeous, golden belt momentarily distracted me. Based on the belt, he could have been heavyweight champion of the world. In an emergency department typically filled with drama, this guy was one cool customer.

What happened to you?

Got gored by a bull.

Pause.

Just as hysteria or an obvious injury can distract from a life threat, so can being stoic. In cases of trauma, we think of the real issue as the "sticker on the forehead." This determines the evaluation and treatment algorithm that needs to be followed. This young man's problem isn't "getting gored by a bull"; it's "penetrating trauma to the abdomen." This could be a life-threatening situation. Even though he's cool and obviously tolerates pain, he could be ready to fall off the proverbial cliff.

The rest of his story was standard fare. He had a laceration to the liver, which is relatively common given the size of the liver. Management of liver injuries has changed in the last twenty-five years. Whereas a generation ago he would have needed an operation, this patient only required admission to the surgical unit, where he had a good recovery. Fortunately, he had no other injuries or complications.

What I remember most about this case and others like it isn't the drama of being gored by a bull. In some ways, that's the same as being stabbed with a dirty knife, which occurs even more often. What stays with me is how wonderfully and curiously diverse we are. I can imagine so many people looking at any of the scenarios—the ice swimmers, the tornado chasers, the cowboys, the pro-gun family members—and immediately turning into judgment mode: "That's ridiculous. Why do people do such things? They're so stupid!"

In fact, this is a huge country, and we would do well to stop pretending that we're a homogenized people. We're amazingly diverse, and it is quite the trick to tolerate each other. Tolerance is the first step before acceptance. Understanding is not required.

All of that being said, I really don't understand the attraction of swimming with sharks . . .

Marbles

Parents have one main job: keep the kids safe, no matter how they otherwise turn out. Never mind that the task is impossible. You have to childproof your house! Infants and children are wired to explore their worlds. They test limits. They'll place anything in their mouths. And they'll put everything in their nose, ears, or wherever else they can. It shouldn't serve as a comfort that in most cases emergency rooms can right some wrongs, because some of the things we have to do to help are just as bad as the problem. A lot of that is because it's the only option available, but sometimes it's due to what happened.

For example, when a kid places a penny or most toys in their nose, surgical clamps can be used to extract it. However, when you have a round, smooth object such as a marble, that can be a lot more difficult to extract. There's a risk of harming the area behind the marble or pushing it down the throat into the windpipe or into the stomach.

I remember the first child I had to treat with a marble stuck in the nose. It's a situation where both you and the nurses are hoping you're lucky, because even with proper technique, you need luck. Questions abound. *Can I do this quickly? Will this kid cooperate? Will I have to strap him down on the papoose board? Will I have to put him to sleep? How do I keep the mother calm? Am I prepared to deal with possible complications?*

Every action taken is an exercise in wistfulness. *I really hope this works, so I don't have to . . .* The efforts involve incrementally more invasive procedures with more risk and a higher probability of being successful. Of course, one could start with the more invasive and definitive option, but you never want to place a child at risk if it can be avoided. And the good news is that the marble always seems to come out (at least, it did for me). I guess when you get rid of the voices and focus on the technique, things work out.

There's nothing better than finishing, grabbing the rescued baby, and handing him or her back to Mom for a big hug. Mothers' intuition is truer than they know. There is a real danger in these things. We just work very hard to make difficult circumstances appear to be a lot easier than they actually are.

Sex and Drugs
in the Hospital

It would shock you to know how often I have stumbled across patients engaging in illicit activity inside of hospitals. I don't know if any phrase has been coined for this activity, but patients seem to pursue it as if it were an item on a "bucket list."

My first experiences with this were the most frightening. I spent a month working the medical floors at a hospital whose reputation for these things was well known. It didn't take long to learn that there was an entire section of the hospital that was understood to be the meeting place for sex and drug use. It was so bad that security officers had to be stationed outside the bathroom. It was so bad that even when you walked past the security officers stationed outside the bathroom and opened the door to the bathroom, you would be greeted with a cloud of smoke. It was common to find needles used for intramuscular injections and multiple items of paraphernalia. It had never occurred to me how easy it would be for visitors or others to engage in drug trafficking inside the walls of a hospital. Was it possible that the security officers were in on it all?

As bad as the drug use was, the sexual activity was even more prevalent. Patients and their visitors routinely were found in bed together. They rarely seemed embarrassed, and they always had the widest grins on their faces. The even more concerning circumstance involved when different patients would end up in bed together. This would include patients with HIV/AIDS and other infectious diseases that were easily transmittable. I would wonder, *What are they thinking?*, but the answer was obvious. Sometimes you forget just how long some of these hospital stays are.

My question was always the same: *What am I supposed to do about this?*

I have never seen a code of conduct for patients who present to hospitals that covers these contingencies. It's a set of tricky ethical questions, though.

- Under what circumstances are you allowed to throw a patient who hasn't fully recovered out of the hospital? How can this ever be justified if doing so would release a communicable disease into the community?
- What is the hospital's recourse if one patient endangers another?
- What is the hospital's liability if a disease is communicated from a sexually transmitted infection or IV drug use while within the hospital?

This type of disregard for public decorum is a fascinating example of human behavior that you would never expect or believe—until you have seen it often enough to not be surprised by it. Lesson learned? Given time, space, and opportunity, many people will do most anything. That lesson gets reinforced again and again with each new patient.

"I Haven't Seen a Doctor in over Forty Years!"

Ugh. That really could be the entire story.

However, this is not that story. You should already know the value of routine preventative care and prompt attention to signs and symptoms as they develop. This story is not about those concerns. This is the story of a decision to live life on one's own terms and a willingness to deal with the consequences of those decisions.

It's a generational thing, or at least, there are those of a certain generation that are more likely to feel this way. There was a time when certain people had a violent fear of doctors and hospitals.

> Go to the hospital? Noooo . . . That's where the diseases are!

This was a tried and true piece of logic. Here's another one:

> The last two times I went to the hospital, someone ended up dying!

Some people are paralyzed into inactivity and over-activity by their fears. We see this in many ways. People fail to get vaccinated. They take multiple vitamins daily for no good reason. They insist on taking antibiotics for colds.

For those who don't pursue routine medical care, it's a dangerous game of chance. However, it does raise a certain question. Would you rather live forty years peacefully before you "crash and burn," or would you want to know as soon as possible what's happening to you, even if its discovery causes you pain and mental anguish?

I have seen several patients who have gone decades without seeing a physician. They always sound so proud about it, as if they have proven they know better. It does raise the issue of the life better lived. This seems like a different version of "live fast, die young," maybe modified to "live oblivious, die whenever."

I remember one "little old lady" who came to the emergency room. She looked me up and down and told me she hadn't seen a doctor in over forty years. She captured so many different sentiments at the same time:

- She was happy that she'd gone forty years without us bothering her.
- She was determined that we get it right, lest she go another forty years without us.
- She was resigned to accept whatever fate befell her.

She displayed an amazing amount of fortitude, and she was very sharp. She looked healthy. Some patients just have good genes, and physicians can tell when this is the case. She was a healthy eater and still did lots of work around the house. Her only issue was that she was a smoker. That's actually why she didn't bother with doctors. She didn't want to hear us running our mouths about her life choices.

The dirty little secret is that sometimes that actually works—if you have great genes and a lot of luck. The problem is that a lot of people are deluded about the probability of them being that person.

This lady ended up being diagnosed with lung cancer.

Sometimes different isn't better or worse; it's just different. The choices we make and the ways we choose to live our lives belong to us and, to a lesser extent, to our families and other loved ones. We just need to learn to make better choices, or at least the best choices for us. We also need to be prepared to live with the full consequences of those choices. Choose well, and live a happy, fulfilled life.

BEHIND THE CURTAIN

At the end of the day, if our choices provide us with a life of happiness, regardless of the ending, would you really argue that the ending invalidated a life subjectively well lived?

Saturday Night
in the Big City

It's Saturday night in the big city. Emergency departments are used to the "Saturday Night Special" variety of patients who are involved in unfortunate situations. There are the suicide attempts. The victims of trauma. Domestic abuse. Sexual assault. And Saturday night brings in a lot of patients who are intoxicated.

If you think emergency rooms are no fun, the emergency department waiting room (or its equivalent) is even worse. With the massive overcrowding of many emergency rooms over the last few decades, many hospitals began engaging in the process of placing patients deemed not to be true emergencies on a stretcher placed in the hallway, in a corner of the emergency room somewhere, or in the waiting room. This practice is also used for such things as allowing intoxicated patients to "sleep it off."

Allow me to introduce you to four separate rules of emergency medicine:

- The change of shift is the most dangerous time in the emergency room.
- Nothing good happens in the waiting room.
- Never get comfortable with a patient who always presents for the same reason.
- Alcoholics fall down and hit their heads.

I came in to work the night shift in my busy inner-city emergency room. Part of our practice is to review all the patients that are being turned over to us. Some physicians like to "run the board" (i.e., discuss the patients at the central station), and others like to visit the patients with the outgoing doctor one by one. I like to do both. This limits surprises and allows the correct environment for the different types of conversations that need to occur.

On this Saturday night, we were overflowing with patients, and there were many patients who had been waiting to be seen for a long time. After sign-out at the Big Board, we went around to introduce me to all of the patients for whom I would be assuming care. Then we got to the hall patients. Tucked away in a corner around the corner was a known alcoholic. He would check himself in from time to time in a way reminiscent of Floyd on the old *Andy Griffith Show*. Each of the physicians had cared for him on multiple occasions.

As we got to the corner around the corner, the patient was still, much as he normally was. The difference was that he wasn't snoring. I shook him. No movement.

When was the last time he was evaluated?

Before waiting for an answer, I directed my physician to get him to the resuscitation room and do what was necessary.

The patient was pronounced dead approximately ten minutes later.

Many of the really bad things that happen to patients don't happen randomly. Patients have risk factors and engage in risky behaviors. Smokers shouldn't be surprised when bronchitis, emphysema, and lung cancer develop. HIV and other sexually transmitted infections develop in those who don't take appropriate precautions prior to engaging in sexual activity. And then there are those who abuse alcohol.

Alcohol abuse contributes to so many medical conditions that questions about recent alcohol intake are among the first questions you ask after greeting certain patients. They develop pancreatitis. They develop gallstones. They crash cars. They develop hepatitis. And they fall down, hit their heads, and develop bleeds inside of their brains that, as things develop, resemble being drunk. Unfortunately, it doesn't stop there, and patients die unless appropriate diligence is maintained in their care. Not all mental-status changes in alcohol abusers are attributable to alcohol intoxication. My colleague learned that the hard way.

Black Toes

The demographics of emergency medicine dictate the types of injuries and illnesses we see. Here are some examples:

- If it's early in the morning, I'm worried about you awakening to discover someone had a stroke or a heart attack overnight.
- If it's between 8:00 to 9:00 a.m. or 3:00 to 4:00 p.m. and I'm working in a trauma center, I'm worried about a kid getting hit by a car.
- If it's Tuesday or Wednesday, I'm expecting to see sexually transmitted infections. (It takes seventy-two hours to incubate what happened on Friday and Saturday nights.)
- If it's Sunday and I'm working in an NFL city, I'm expecting it to be slow during the game and extremely busy right after the game. There may be alcohol involved.
- If it's November or December, I'm expecting an onslaught of the flu and other respiratory illness.
- If it's the weekend in the summer, I'm expecting trauma.

And on and on. I could write a book about it . . .

So on an otherwise routine middle-of-the-night shift in the dead cold of a winter storm, when the squawk box goes off, I have a pretty good idea what to expect.

> We have a sixty-year-old man found down in a snow bank. He's groggy but easily arousable. There appears to be EtOH (alcohol) involved.

Sometimes when a patient hits the door, you just know. To an extent not seen in other medical specialties, emergency physicians engage in the art of "picture diagnoses." Everything about you is telling me the story of you. Even as I say hello and ask you how you are doing, I'm evaluating your ability to talk, the quality of your voice, and your breathing pattern. The quality of your skin, hair, and nails is easily assessed visually. Of course, once you're undressed, even more information is obtainable. Add all of that to your chief complaint, information that may have been given to me by the paramedics, and what they see (including your vital signs) when you are connected to the heart monitors. In many instances, I already know your story and, to a certain degree, your emergency room course, assessment, and treatment needs, as well as your likely outcome before you have even hit the door. That leaves our conversation to fill in details and verify initial suspicions. This dramatically reduces the time it takes for us to start addressing some emergencies that may exist.

Now, if you're wondering how this is possible, the answer is twofold. The easy answer is that this displays why emergency medicine is a specialty instead of an extension of your primary care doctor's office. This level of awareness is similarly displayed in other professions, such as the instinctual activities of a pilot navigating a plane through trouble. The other consideration is found in the nature of emergency medicine. We're in the primary business of ruling out life threats more than making diagnoses of chronic diseases. Life-threatening conditions converge into common pathways and produce certain reactions within the body, known as clinical signs and symptoms. You not only tell us these things verbally. Your body also speaks for you.

So in the dead middle of winter when you find yourself stranded in a freezing cold, windy environment, or if you're an ice fisherman or similar type of cold-weather thrill seeker, that by itself tells a certain story. When you come in to the emergency department, and, upon undressing you and taking your vital signs, we discover that your temperature is ninety-two degrees and you have black toes, you'll excuse me if I momentarily place a lower priority on removing the splinter in your finger you obtained while falling, even though that's what hurts the most.

Hypothermia (low body temperature) and frostbite are twin life-threatening dangers within the spectrum of cold exposure. Our current patient has several risk factors for hypothermia, and his life is in danger. He's weak, drowsy, and confused, and he is shivering. He displays a low heart rate, and his breathing is slow.

The most important thing regarding his immediate outcome is what's not there. We don't see any evidence that his heart is displaying abnormal activity, and he is still able to maintain his ability to breathe. However, his blood pressure is low, so we are going to deal with that, as well as raise his core body temperature and address his black toes as priorities.

That requires work on several levels at the same time. We have a call into the orthopedic surgeon, who will want to deal with the toes. We initially have the patient undressed, out of his soggy clothes, and covered with warm blankets; this gets replaced with a special warming apparatus. He has hot water bottles placed to his groin, armpits, and both sides of his neck. He's receiving warm oxygen through his nose and warmed IV fluids. These actions are necessary to prevent the type of cold-induced damage that ends a life and serves to rapidly yet safely raise his core body temperature into a safe area.

About those toes . . . They're bathing in a warm whirlpool (actually it's more like hot; the temperature is set at 104 degrees). I notice he has blood blisters on several of the toes. *This isn't good.*

This patient wasn't homeless. He had a home and family. Frostbite can occur to anyone when the circumstances permit. Risky behavior doesn't know the background of the person involved and doesn't care who is affected.

Fast forward: The patient survived. He was admitted to the hospital. His family was discovered. A few months down the road, he had several toes amputated. It was all too predictable.

Why Do You Have
Gonorrhea in Your Eye?

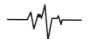

It's not always the things you do that get you in trouble. Sometimes it's the things you don't do. Like wash your hands. Yes. The simplest of activities protects you in ways you never even realize.

In walks a young man into my busy emergency room. The first thing I notice is he can't keep his hands out of his eyes. As often occurs with presentations relating to sexually transmitted infections, the young man has been less than truthful to the female nurses, telling them he had something in his eye. Boy, did he.

He immediately asks the nurses to leave so he can talk to me "man to man." Everyone immediately knows what that means. On the way out, the nurse gives a smirk like the one you give a prepubescent male who suddenly learns modesty.

I already have this figured out. I'm busy, so I cut to the chase. Normally decorum involves a certain bedside manner, but he asked for "man talk."

How long have you had a discharge coming from your penis?

Wow, Doc. How did you know?

Thanks for the compliment. That's why you came to see me, right? How long?

About two weeks.

I'm really surprised it took you that long to come see me. Most men are a little more protective of their privates when stuff happens to them.

Yeah. I thought it would get better.

What about your sexual partners? How many do you have? Do they know about this?

Yeah. One of them did this to me. They're all getting treated.

No. No one "did this to you." You have to accept responsibility for your own actions and your own genitals. What do you think is going on with your eye?

I don't know. My kids at home are sick. I figured it was pink eye.

Don't you think that's a whole lot of stuff coming out of your eye for pink eye?

I noticed that, too. It's really itchy.

OK, let's examine you and run some tests. I will get you taken care of . . .

After the requisite examination, swabs, needles, and blood tests, we're back together.

OK. We have good news and bad news. The good news is that you'll be treated when you leave here, for the most part. We'll keep you on medicine for your eyes.

Then I told him he had gonorrhea. Then I told him the discharge coming from his eye was also from gonorrhea. Then I saw the young man realize he wasn't invincible as he slumped to the chair like a man three times his age.

Gonorrhea is no fun for men. Unlike many sexually transmitted infections, the symptoms in gonorrhea tend to be worse in men than in women. Even though some men don't develop symptoms, when they do, it's not pleasant. There's the burning that occurs with urination. Swollen testes can occur. Rectal infections can cause itching, soreness, bleeding, and difficulty with bowel movements. Away from the genitalia, gonorrhea can cause a sore throat and is notable for copious discharge from the eye.

How does this occur, you may ask? At the end of the day, it involves failure to wash your hands. The process involves jock itch or other reasons to handle your genitals, followed by putting your hands on your face before thoroughly cleaning them. Yes. Please do grimace. It happens more than you think.

As my patient left the emergency room, he slunk out much in the way he had slunk in. Hopefully, the subsequent, more serious conversation we had led him to adapt his behavior.

That's Not a Cold

Trauma patients invariably underestimate the seriousness of the injuries that they suffer and the consequences of actions taken during fights or whatever caused the injury. You can't just punch a wall or put your hand through a plate of glass and then be surprised if surgery is necessary. If you meant to break your hand or slice a tendon, this is what you would have done. You can't brush it off when someone swings a baseball bat at you and it connects with your back. Baseball bats are usually swung with dangerous intentions. Being pistol-whipped, particularly to the head, is going to have consequences. Parts of you are going to break.

When the squawk box sounds off and the paramedics tell us they have "a young male, BHT with LOC (blunt head trauma with loss of consciousness)," anything could be happening. By the time this patient arrived to the emergency department, he was wearing a *cervical collar* (hard neck brace) and was strapped onto a backboard.

When people talk about having concussions, does that actually register with you? Even now, we have taken to treating concussions like they're bad ankle sprains. "If he passes the neurological testing, he'll be allowed to return to the game . . ."

No.

A concussion is a symptom of a traumatic brain injury, recognized by symptoms such as loss of consciousness, altered mental status, or a significant headache. Allow me to focus on the important part of that sentence: *Traumatic. Brain. Injury.* You have only one brain, and if it's injured, it's not going to heal itself. The point is that an injury that produces a concussion needs to be identified, instead of attempting to prove that it's OK to return to the same conditions that produced the injury.

The young man looks bad. He's beat up and has bruises all about his head and neck, including behind his ears. He has black eyes that are so discolored that he looks like a raccoon. He is sore and tender at multiple parts of his body, including bruising to his back and deformed forearms, presumably from blocking the assault with the baseball bats. Apparently, after he blacked out, his multiple assailants continued to deliver whatever message they felt needed to be sent.

As multiple actions are occurring simultaneously, I notice the presence of clear fluid coming from his nose.

Have you had a cold lately?

Actually I have. Why do you ask?

Have you had any drainage from your nose?

Not really. I have been sniffing and coughing some.

I immediately wonder what would have happened to this patient if he hadn't received transportation to the emergency department and had the same level of injuries, but only to the head. Likely he would have taken some pain medications and waited it out. He would have interpreted his nasal drainage as part of his evolving cold symptoms.

This patient has a fracture to the bones at the base of his brain, known as a basilar skull fracture, and additionally has assorted broken bones in his extremities. He is also found to have significant bruising to his kidneys—he actually has a substantial amount of blood in his urine.

Regarding the head injuries, the patient required only close observation in the hospital. Had he stayed home, the upper respiratory tract infection could have found its way to the brain, causing a dramatic infection to accompany the injuries.

Don't make the mistake of thinking that because sometimes things work out OK, they were supposed to. This type of story with a good outcome is the exception, not the rule. A good rule of thumb for any victim of trauma is "It's better to have received a medical clearance exam that seemed like a waste of time than to have needed one and not gotten it."

"Doc, If I Don't Hold My Head, It'll Fall Off!"

There are some things that patients say to you that seem to make no sense—at least the first time you hear them. This is one of them. By the way, he was telling the truth.

Now, how would you respond if someone came running into your office (in my case, the emergency room) saying that? I know, right? Well, in my business, there's plenty of time to get the psychiatrists involved if and when it's needed, but emergency medicine is about ruling out life threats, and as luck would have it, there's a situation in which such a claim is actually correct. Besides, haven't you ever wondered exactly how your head sits and stays on top of your body?

So this middle-aged, intoxicated gentleman comes into the emergency room via ambulance (and thank goodness I'm working at a level 1 trauma center, which means it's equipped for everything). He won't stop screaming about his head, which he believes snapped after a motor vehicle collision (they're not accidents). His examination reveals paralysis of his legs, increased reflexes, and decreased ability to grasp objects. In these circumstances, even before arrival, the paramedics have stabilized the neck with a *hard cervical brace* (a.k.a., a C-collar).

As an emergency physician, no matter how seemingly outlandish the claim, my first response is always to listen and consider the validity of what a patient is telling me. Too often, serious conditions have a time component to treatment, and any time wasted decreases the probability of a successful outcome.

This case was actually easier than other, similar ones because the patient had additional, definite findings indicating the nervous symptom was damaged.

The injury this patient suffered is called a *bilateral facet dislocation*. The facet joints are the structures that connect the *vertebrae* (the bones in your spine) to each other. Fractures, dislocations, and disruptions to the ligaments that combine to keep everything in place can lead to an unstable head and neck. In this type of injury to the neck, it doesn't take much to imagine the cervical (neck) vertebrae nearly completely displaced from the one below it.

If you think it's easy to think about all this in the midst of a loud, drunk, malodorous patient, you would be wrong. It's challenging not to ascribe it all to the ranting of an intoxicated man. Obviously, that would be a mistake.

Next stop is a visit to the neurosurgeon. Believe it or not, the patient ended up OK, relatively speaking. I felt great about the save, but I would have felt even better if he had agreed to stop drinking.

"Doc, My Breath Smells Like *!?#$%"

What do you say to a guy who says this? Is this a cry for help for really, really bad breath? Is it possible that he got *!?#$% in his mouth?

There are things patients say to you that are buzzwords for certain medical conditions. For example, if you tell me your child is barking like a seal, I'm concerned about *croup*. If you tell me your jaw is clicking when you open and close it, I'm thinking about *TMJ disorder* (temporomandibular joint). If you tell me you see halos, I would be concerned about *glaucoma* or perhaps *digoxin toxicity* (if you take that drug). If a young lady expresses concern about a fishy odor, I think about *BV* (bacterial vaginosis). There are many, many examples of this, including when your breath smells like feces or you have the taste of feces in your mouth.

This poor gentleman came into the emergency department looking sick and feeling sicker. Imagine feeling sick to your stomach from the smell of feces but not being able to stop vomiting. Throw in some abdominal pain and distention, and you have the picture of this very unhappy man.

This is also an example of a disconnect in priorities between doctor and patient. Place yourself in his shoes. I'm pretty sure that you would say that no matter what else you're feeling, getting that taste out of your mouth is going to be a pretty high priority. All things considered, that wasn't even on my radar initially because that symptom is not itself a life threat. That's not being insensitive; it's just how things had to be prioritized, because something serious actually was occurring.

This patient's presentation, diagnosis, and bizz-buzz were consistent with a condition known as a *small bowel obstruction*. The general problem is that at some level of your intestines (which is absorbing your digested food and transporting your undigested food through to be excreted as feces), things have become blocked. Your body can hold only so much, and the contents of the stomach and intestines need a way out. If they can't come out the back end, sometimes vomiting will ensue and contents will come back out of your mouth. The notion of the smell and taste of feces was an accurate assessment of what was occurring. If this condition doesn't get resolved, it can become an emergency that requires surgery.

In case you're wondering what's done about this, the simple answer is that the bowel needs to be placed at rest and emptied. That means you don't get to put any more food in your mouth, and one of those annoying rubber tubes gets placed through your nose, down your throat, and into your stomach to evacuate its contents.

As onerous as this sounds, the patient didn't seem to mind. Once the immediate threat was addressed, we got him some medical mouthwash, and I think he was sufficiently distracted by the tube in his nose.

The next time something seemingly esoteric happens to you like the sensation of a lightning bolt running through your face or a reversal of hot and cold sensations, don't ignore it. It may actually be something significant.

Saving the Family Jewels

No, this is not a story about a heroic patient who battled a would-be burglar. This is a story that illustrates a very important Rule of Emergency Medicine:

Time Is Tissue.

Sometimes internal defense mechanisms can actually confuse the body and/or physicians providing care for patients. Many examples of this exist in our immune system's responses to our own bodies (called *autoimmune diseases*). The pain a man experiences when having some insult or injury to the groin is not on that list. That pain serves men well because it sends a message that is directly in line with the reality of the matter: *this needs to be seen by a physician*.

In one common instance of such pain, a young male on the verge of puberty presents with acute pain to one of his testicles. Unlike other problems to the area, such as rashes and discharge from the penis that could be from a sexually transmitted infection, these patients aren't whispering. They're either sobbing or yelling, but they're definitely in pain.

This is another example of when it's the wrong move for the emergency physician to spend a lot of time in conversation, although some information is vital. There's a future-ability-to-create-life, as well as a life-threatening condition, that needs to be ruled out called testicular torsion. The torsion is a twisting of a portion of the scrotum (the spermatic cord) that chokes off blood supply to the testes and other portions of the scrotum. If this problem is satisfactorily addressed within six hours, the testicle can be saved. If not, the risk of losing function and the testicle itself dramatically and incrementally increases due to the consequences of the reduced blood flow.

The urgency of the matter is the predominant thought going through my mind. These concerns need to be communicated in a way to help the family understand that I'm not displaying a lack of interest in talking to the family or the child. I also don't want them to get the impression that I just want to start manipulating his genitals, as it's extremely likely that these typically young males may not be used to such aggressive maneuvers. That part isn't so hard. Parents are usually impressed with a lot of hurried activity, and, in this example, a lot is being mobilized at once. The radiology department is being notified to get testing done as soon as possible that can confirm the diagnosis. Perhaps the genital/urinary surgeon is being notified of a possible case. There are other tests that need to be done as well. Additionally, I need to make an effort to manually reverse the torsion if that is high on the list of possible causes of this testicular pain.

Manual detorsion is the name for the medical procedure that reverses the twisting of the testicle. It basically involves a motion similar to opening and closing a book (don't try this at home). The premise is that the twisting of the cord predominantly occurs in one direction and it might be amenable to manual reversal. If and when this premise is correct, the reversal will bring significant relief of pain and probable improvement of blood flow. Of course, the situation can also be made worse.

I'm pleased to say that in every case I have ever seen, the outcome was reducible to one variable: the time from when the symptoms started to when they came in for evaluation. As mentioned, when evaluation occurs within six hours, a good outcome can be produced. Although many cases can't be prevented, those occurring due to injury need to be seen promptly. This is not something you want to wait a day to see if it will "get better on its own." The fate of generations could be hinging on the decision you make.

You Didn't Realize You
Left That There?

Shock is a severe situation involving disruption of several of the body's functions. Whether or not it's due to infection, your life hangs in the balance. Shock isn't a symptom; it's the intersection of multiple potentially disastrous events. When shock occurs in a younger individual, it gives you pause. Younger individuals are more resilient and better able to ward off illness. When shock sets in, that could be an indicator of some compromise within the individual's immunity or just a measure of how ferocious the cause of the shock is.

Into a busy emergency department rolls an obviously ill young woman in her twenties. Her family notes she hasn't been seen in the last week and is now much less responsive than normal. The patient is confused and very hot. She smells like stool and blood and is covered in a fine red rash. Her blood pressure is very low, and her heart rate is very fast. She looks ill.

It's an important process in the emergency department that the diagnosis isn't as important as addressing the life threats (even though patients seem to want to know "what's wrong" as soon as they walk in the door). Even as we focus on the three or four most likely considerations and consequently rule out each of them, the primary concern remains addressing what's trying to kill you; we'll deal with the actual diagnosis in due time. In this case, it is probable that a massive infection is present. Because of the severity of the symptoms, this isn't just any infection. This is a big one, on the order of meningitis or encephalitis—there aren't many infections that just overwhelm young, healthy individuals.

As blood tests and emergency treatment measures such as IV fluids, prophylactic antibiotics, and medicine to bring down the fever are given, it's time to analyze the clues. In life-threatening situations, sometimes it's more important to shoot first and ask questions later, but it is important to ask questions. When a patient is confused and minimally responsive, he or she communicates through physical symptoms. The physical exam becomes very important.

We're scrambling for a source of infection.

> We know the patient smells of blood and stools, so that's one clue. The ears are clear. The nose doesn't have any discharge. The throat isn't red. The neck isn't stiff. The lungs are surprisingly clear. The patient does have a fine red rash but nothing that looks like a skin infection. Hmm . . .

> How about these stools. Wait; compressing the lower portion of the belly makes the patient moan. It could be a urinary tract infection that has spread throughout the body, but that tends to happen in patients a lot older than this, and she's otherwise healthy. Let's look at the stools.

> Well, the stool is what I would expect for diarrhea. It doesn't have the smell or other features of things that fit this picture. But . . .

> That smell of blood isn't coming from the stools; it's coming from the vagina. Might she have a fistula? (A fistula is an abnormal communication between two structures. They tend to occur from surgeries, infections, or other injuries. If that was the case here, stool might be coming through the vagina.) She'll need a pelvic examination.

It's a diagnostic dilemma when there is the simultaneous presence of blood and diarrhea below the waist. It could represent bloody diarrhea or the presence of menstrual blood and diarrhea separately. The diarrhea could be a disease unto itself or part of a loss of bodily functions. In any event, the combination requires evaluation.

We clean the patient up, get her ready for the exam, I place the speculum in, and . . .

Whoa. What is that smell?

Can you imagine a smell so bad that it overpowers the smell of diarrhea? I actually checked to make sure I was wearing a mask (I was). Well, I can, and it instantly brings a consideration to the top of the list of possibilities.

Toxic shock syndrome (TSS) is an illness that is caused by infection with a specific bacteria named *staphylococcus* (perhaps you know it as "staph"; those famous MRSA—methicillin-resistant staph aureus—skin infections are also caused by it). The problem is that infections aren't just limited to the site where the bacteria exists. It releases toxins that spread throughout the body. TSS was once overwhelmingly associated with packings such as those that are placed in your nose to stop bleeding, but especially with tampon use—particularly if you inadvertently leave it in and/or forget it's there. TSS causes disruption, if not outright failure, of several of the body's organs, most notably the kidneys. TSS may be fatal in up to 50 percent of cases.

The examination on my patient did reveal a tampon, which was removed. After a prolonged stay in the Intensive Care Unit, antibiotics, and other supportive measures, she made a full recovery.

I don't believe I ever saw this patient again. If I did, I don't even know that I would recognize her. That's too bad. It's amazing that you can have such an impact on someone's life and remain anonymous. Oh well. At least there's solace in knowing the impact was made.

I'm Hanging Out

There are all kinds of things that happen to people that never get discussed in polite company. However, you have heard about them, haven't you? Doctors and nurses in an emergency room think about these things when people display certain tell-tale signs. One of those signs is a person's walk. I'm not talking about the type of walk someone has with a hip replacement or a prosthesis placed after a foot or leg amputation. I'm describing the walk that tells you something bad just happened. Have you ever heard of the *PID* (pelvic inflammatory disease) shuffle? That's one, and some of you know exactly what I mean. Well, there's more. Patients who have active ulcers or sores—say, from either an abscess (you call them boils) or an active herpes infection—also walk in a way that minimizes skin contact.

I remember the first time I saw a certain type of walk that I hadn't previously. This was an elderly patient who was hunched over, walking very slowly with her legs held very closely together while escorted by her daughter. She held her arms shyly on the top of her thighs. We rushed to get her a wheelchair and placed her in a room.

She got straight to the point. "Doc, please help me. I don't know what happened, but something's hanging out of me as if I'm having a baby!"

She was approximately seventy, so I was pretty sure that wasn't the case. However, she could have been thirty with the same story.

The patient was describing a *uterine prolapse*. The uterus (womb) is supported by a variety of muscles on the floor of your pelvis. These muscles very nicely cradle the uterus and other pelvic organs, such as your bladder and bowel, keeping everything in place and functioning normally. With age and even more so with pregnancy and childbirth, the support mechanism can become damaged or weakened enough that the uterus will protrude through the vagina.

The patient was deathly afraid of coughing or having other parts of her falling out or apart. Fortunately, the process to return the uterus back to its normal position is pretty straightforward. In terms of what happens next, Kegel exercises are a great means of strengthening the pelvic muscles. In some instances, a removable medical device called a *pessary* can be placed in the vagina to support the involved organs. She did well.

It is a weird happenstance of the emergency department that certain days seem to have themes. It really isn't uncommon to see multiple patients with the same diagnosis or a variation of the same theme in the same day. And so it was on this day.

Later in the same day, a thin, elderly gentleman came to the emergency department. He also had a waddle, but his was slightly different. He had an upright stance, but he was nearly bent over backwards (well, as much as he could be). He had his hands on his buttocks as he took slow, steady steps.

I look at my nurse, who has grabbed a stretcher and glances back at me, smiling. *Good choice not getting a wheelchair*, I nod back at her.

This didn't take long.

> Doc, I've been constipated a lot. I was straining to help pass a stool, and the next thing I know, I'm feeling a lot of pressure and pain.

Examination reveals that this gentleman has a *prolapsed rectum*. All joking aside, the reddish structure coming out of the rectum resembled the type of aliens that have protruded from the bodies of various characters in several movies.

The process of reducing the prolapsed rectum is simple and similar to addressing the prolapsed uterus. There is one additional point of interest worth mentioning. Placement of simple table sugar or salt has been shown to decrease swelling and facilitate spontaneous reduction of the mass back into place (don't try this at home).

Fortunately, this gentleman responded well. Had that not been the case, surgery likely would have been required. In case you were wondering, this happens even more frequently in children younger than age six.

When the day is over and you find yourself outside the hospital, if you have any hopes of having a normal life and any sense of mental stability, it becomes important to place certain events of the day in the trash can of your memory. Little does anyone at home know that I have spent a significant part of my day placing unmentionables back where they're supposed to be. That's probably a good thing.

The fight for normalcy continues.

Why Some Doctors Won't Shake Your Hand

It's pretty amazing how much danger physicians, nurses, and other members of the hospital staff place themselves in. In addition to increased rates of suicide, substance abuse, divorce, and a decreased life expectancy, physicians are exposed to HIV and hepatitis from needle sticks and blood exposure as well as multiple forms of life-threatening infectious diseases, including meningitis, pneumonia, tuberculosis, and others, all obtained from breathing the same air as our patients or coming into contact in the ways necessary to do our jobs. Of course, there are precautions that we take to minimize those risks, but they're still there.

The dangers are real, and not just in the ways I have described already. Here are two examples of how the simple act of the most common of courtesies—shaking hands—has gotten colleagues of mine exposed in a way that no worker should.

Several rashes appear on the palms of your hands and the soles of your feet. The one most applicable here is the second stage of syphilis. It's a rather nondescript rash, but under the right (read: wrong) circumstances, there it is, and it can be transmitted.

Similarly, there's a sore that can appear on the hand that can easily be confused for a *pustule* (pus bump), or other types of infections of the fingers, including those called *paronychiae* or *felons*. Unfortunately, there's a similarly appearing infection caused by herpes simplex virus called *herpetic whitlow*.

So please don't take offense if your doctor walks into the room on occasion (typically this will occur based on your presenting concern) wearing a mask or gloves or if you have a rash and he or she declines the usual handshake prior to a complete examination. On the other hand (no pun intended), have you ever noticed whether your emergency room doctors and nurses wash their hands before and/or after they leave the room? You deserve protection as well.

In fact, you'd do well to adopt this posture yourself. You're always bringing friends, family, and loved ones to the emergency room for evaluation of rashes. Rashes in unusual locations or even in usual locations, such as the genitals, should really prompt a hard stop of whatever you're doing and a prompt trip in for evaluation. Caution is a better course of action than regret.

Spinal Tap

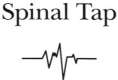

I had a college student come into the emergency department one day whom I recognized because I had cared for her on a few occasions. Although she typically was very chipper and smiling, today she was not. As she sauntered by to her room, I noticed that she was walking as you might imagine a mummy or Frankenstein would, meaning everything was straight ahead, military march, with her head locked in place. As I called out to say hello, she had to turn her entire body. She chose not to move her neck. I looked at my nurse, and she nodded "yes." I yelled at her to put on a mask.

The patient had a fever that started quickly and a massive headache. She reported that there had been an outbreak of meningitis on campus. Her examination revealed all the classic signs. Most notably, when I attempted to bend her neck forward with my hand on the back of her head, I ended up lifting her chest off the table. That's called *nuchal rigidity*, and it's a clear sign that she's probably infected.

Meningitis is the inflammation of the layer of tissue surrounding the brain and spinal cord. Viruses are the most common cause of meningitis, but when caused by bacteria, it is life-threatening and can leave you with a stroke and brain damage.

One particular problem with meningitis is how rapidly it spreads. Thus, when symptoms start and you get to the emergency room, we get straight to work. After doing appropriate testing, we need to obtain a lumbar puncture (a.k.a., spinal tap).

Spinal taps are somewhat legendary in popular culture; there's even a heavy metal band with the name, as well as a movie. I think this has added to the drama surrounding the procedure. A spinal tap is a medical procedure performed to extract *cerebrospinal fluid* (CSF—the naturally occurring fluid that bathes the spinal cord) from the spinal column, the bones in your back. A special spinal needle is used to maneuver between the bones and enter the spinal column. Sufficient fluid is drained to run the tests necessary to determine if and which type of infection is present. There are risks, including bleeding, pain, and even paralysis (although I have never seen or heard of anyone who knows anyone in whom this has happened). Regarding the pain, you get local anesthesia (numbing medicine) beforehand, so the pain ends up being similar to getting an IV started, unless the doctor takes the needle too far into the spinal column and strikes some of the nerves in the spinal cord. Overall, it's actually a very safe procedure in experienced hands.

Fortunately, this patient tolerated the procedure well. In fact, we accomplished what we call a *Champagne Tap*, one in which no blood cells are obtained (back in residency training, if you performed the procedure and did this, someone owed you a bottle of champagne). This is important because blood cells can actually distort the results. The results came back, and she was diagnosed with viral meningitis.

Patients get so frustrated when they have a diagnosis (especially a serious diagnosis such as meningitis) and you tell them that there is nothing to do other than supportive measures. For future reference, whenever you hear the words "virus" or "viral," generally expect the conversation to turn toward "You're going home. Rest, drink plenty of fluids, and you won't be receiving any antibiotics." Intuitively, that makes no sense for something this serious, but most people (i.e., those with normally functioning immune systems) will have a complete recovery in seven to ten days. In the case of our patient, she was made to feel much better after one or two hours of supportive treatment, and she went home.

The very next day, the patient came back. Her neck was already starting to get better, but the issue today was her headache. It was even worse than before and had become unbearable.

After proper evaluation and having excluded other considerations, it was apparent that this was a *spinal headache*. A spinal headache is another complication of a lumbar puncture. It results from leakage of spinal fluid from the spinal column after the lumbar puncture. The risks of this occurring increase if the patient doesn't rest or assume the appropriate position (flat on the back for about two hours) after completion of the procedure. Larger needle sizes also increase the risk.

As mentioned, this complication results from a leak in the spinal column that resulted from the lumbar puncture. The treatment involves patching that leak. This is done by drawing blood from the patient then taking that blood and inserting it into the spot where the spinal tap occurred. That's right. The patient required another spinal tap, except in this case she needed blood inserted into the space inside instead of having fluid extracted.

She was also given pain medication and felt better before too long. She again returned home, and on the next occasion that I saw her (for a problem involving her mother), she was back to being the buoyant, delightful young lady to whom I enjoyed providing care. Medical care works. I'm glad she got to us early.

Angel Dusted Off

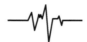

From the department of déjà vu all over again (with apologies to the great Baseball Hall of Famer Yogi Berra), I had reason to reflect on nearly identical presentations that occurred nearly twenty years apart.

Both patients were young, male, wildly hallucinating, out of control, and strong as an ox. Twenty years ago, such patients were gang-tackled and placed in leather restraints; that doesn't occur so much anymore. Even after being restrained, they each managed to lift up the bed and flip it, while still in it. Next, after the restraints were tightened, they both dislocated their shoulders trying to get out of them. Both of these patients received so much sedation that I thought I was going to have to treat them for a second overdose.

Despite the apparent appeal of the hallucinations and psychotic episodes, PCP went out of style in the 1990s with the emergence of other, easier, and less dramatic ways to get high. Then a few short years ago, PCP began to make a comeback. Now, it's all about getting "wet." PCP is Angel Dust no more. The new formulation of PCP involves dissolving it in fluid, followed by soaking cigarettes in the fluid and smoking once dry. These are called "dippers."

Of all the illicit drugs people take, PCP has always been the most curious to me. For those deciding to take the drug for the first time, the notion that you actually would want to dissociate from reality is an act akin to wanting to commit suicide. Basically, you're saying you don't want to be here. For those who are repeaters, it's even more shocking. I have never seen anyone on PCP have a "good trip." They are in a state that closely resembles schizophrenia, from our viewpoint. What's happening on the other side of reality must be amazing. I actually recall an additional patient who mentally had stepped outside of himself and was engaging himself as if he now had a twin. Now, that's tripping.

Both of my patients, and PCP users in general, are signing up to take a leap off a building, both figuratively and, in several documented instances, literally. These patients are completely out of touch with reality. They place themselves in harm's way in several different ways. No one comes into an emergency department on PCP and just waits it out. Whatever medical issues exist, medical providers find these patients very difficult to diagnose, as they are either ragingly psychotic or completely detached. In whichever circumstance, they're not providing a medical history about their problems. These patients can remain comatose and catatonic for days. Some patients continue to have psychotic episodes long after stopping the drug. Taking PCP means "Coming soon to a psychiatric hospital near you."

Is there a lesson to be had in patients intoxicated by PCP? I hope you will appreciate the gravity of the conditions leading to wanting to dissociate from reality. There is an abundance of help available to you, even if it doesn't seem like it at any single point in time that you happen to be in immediate duress. Perhaps one should also learn that there are some actions beyond which there's no point of return.

Fight and Flight Risks

Consider the following stories. What do these patients have in common?

- The police bring a suspect to the emergency department for blood alcohol testing and medical clearance. Once the medical clearance is done, he'll be taken to jail. While waiting in the emergency department, the police respond to a disturbance elsewhere in the department.
- A patient is brought into the emergency department after a heroin overdose. His overdose is reversed with appropriate medication. He has a warrant out for his arrest.
- A seventeen-year-old female is brought to the emergency department after a suicide attempt. She continually claims she did it because she was trying to get attention from her boyfriend, who has just broken up with her. Despite this, the decision has been made to transport her to an inpatient psychiatric facility.

These three patients each made a run for it. They identified themselves as destined for a place they really didn't want to be, knew they had someone coming for them, and decided to take their chances.

Now, consider these additional three stories. Can you guess what these patients had in common?

- An IV drug addict has been in the emergency department for several hours. He's craving his next fix. He takes advantage of a lull in the department and escapes. He returns two hours later obviously high. The IV that was placed in the emergency department is still in place but apparently was used as the route of drug delivery for his most recent injection.
- A female comes to the emergency department with multiple bruises. Her male companion comes in and begins to beat on her.
- A patient is brought to the emergency department after attempting suicide. He grabs a piece of equipment within the room and proceeds to commit additional harm.

Occasionally, patients are in danger from themselves or others while in the emergency department. In most instances, the emergency department staff lacks the training and authority to intervene physically in these types of situations.

Here is a final set of three stories:

- A patient is in the emergency department after a gang fight. He believes the opposing gang members are going to come for him. He wants to leave. The staff tells him he can't leave.
- A patient is in the emergency department after getting high on unknown substances, possibly including cocaine and PCP. He believes he recognizes a staff member as someone who's "out to get him."
- A patient is a frequent visitor to the emergency department and is thought to be a drug seeker. After receiving a medical clearance exam, the staff tells him that he is being discharged and will not be receiving any prescriptions for outpatient narcotics.

These three patients went on to either physically intimidate or attack various members of the emergency department staff.

You probably take for granted that you and your family are secure while you're in the emergency department. For the most part, you are. On the other hand, it takes only one bad episode to change someone's life for the worse.

The emergency department and hospital staffs are placed in all kinds of physical danger without any direct means of defense. I actually sat in my office while a nurse was being murdered exactly one floor below me (the story made front page national news; I was unaware of the occurrence while it was happening). Since then, several things have changed regarding hospital security. Emergency departments have become closed units. Metal detectors are common in large trauma centers. Many emergency departments have security forces. Yet still others don't, and they depend on an assortment of males otherwise staffing the hospital to respond to a special code designed to be a cry for help. Other hospitals leave their staff waiting for the local police department to show.

It's hard to believe that either patients or staff would be put in such a position in this day and age. One would think that after the types of assaults and even deaths that have occurred—both to patients and staff—that emergency departments across the country would be required to have a security presence. The time for you to find out the security policies of your favorite hospital is well before you find yourself in a skirmish. Ask.

You Blew My High!

A patient with an altered mental status is a scary proposition on the face of it. You don't know what's occurring. It could be a coma, or the patient could be suffering from some brain injury, from meningitis, or from the effects of alcohol intoxication or be in the midst of a heart attack or a stroke. Alternatively, it could be something like an excessively high or low glucose (i.e., blood sugar) level or a disruption in oxygen levels. In any event, when the patient has a severe enough set of circumstances that brain function is even temporarily disrupted, it is a medical emergency.

Years and years ago, I learned how to administer what was called a *Coma Cocktail* to patients who came into the emergency department with altered mental statuses. This combination of medicines plus an accompanying algorithm of tests and procedures was designed to cover a broad array of conditions and potential life threats.

From the department of unintended consequences comes a story of treatment that worked too well. The paramedics bring in a young, seemingly healthy patient who appears to be sleeping pretty deeply, at least if his snoring is any indication. A physical examination reveals telltale signs including pupils that had become pinpoint in size, a labored breathing pattern, and the presence of track marks (needle sticks indicating IV drug use).

One thing that is true in emergency medicine is that you can't be distracted by the obvious. Even as we had this part of the puzzle figured out, the search continued for other life-threatening conditions. For example, there's nothing preventing a guy who overdosed on heroin from also being struck upside the head with the butt of a gun after a bad drug deal. Once we were convinced that nothing else was of a higher priority than his probable heroin overdose, and we had gotten to a certain point in the treatment algorithm, we gave him a medication used to reverse the effects of heroin.

The medicine works. The patient sits up, looks around, sizes up the situation, and snarls at us, "You blew my high!" He rips out his IV from his arm, takes the oxygen tubing away from his nose, jumps off the stretcher, and runs out of the emergency department.

As the staff sits there stunned, there are a few questions and issues needing to be addressed:

- First and foremost, the staff is not going to place themselves at harm chasing a patient under the influence of drugs. If he gets up and runs away, unless security can intervene, he's gone.
- Also, this gentleman could be in danger. Neither his medical evaluation nor his treatment has been completed. The police need to be contacted to find this patient.

Approximately an hour later, the patient is again brought back by ambulance. The police had located him back in the same condition as when I first saw him.

We have "treatment amnesia" about some things in the emergency room. This second presentation cannot be treated as an extension of the first. The patient could have done different drugs, received trauma, or had a stroke since the first episode. So we start from scratch. Luckily, the circumstances are the same except for one difference—we didn't forget everything (meaning we now knew he was a flight risk). This time we place restraints on his arms and legs so he can't escape (he's actually in police custody at this point anyway). This time when he awakens, he just starts cursing, which calms down once the police get involved.

It takes just under an hour for the various new tests to come back. It looks like a simple heroin overdose (or at least some member of the opiate narcotic family). Going back into the room to reevaluate him, I discover that he has yet again passed out.

Sigh. We're fortunate to have completed our workup at this point, because the answer to this riddle is pretty straightforward. The medicine being used to reverse the narcotic has a shorter half-life (i.e., duration of action) than the narcotic itself. This means that as the reversal agent wears off, the narcotic will again take effect. Given the specific drug and the double dosing the patient engaged in, this could take a while. He ends up needing to be admitted to the hospital.

Things have changed a bit since then. Paramedics are now able to administer this medicine on the ambulance prior to arrival in the emergency room, so the issue about the mystery of heroin overdose is already cleared from consideration. Also, the use of physical restraints has been dramatically restricted. However, this case dramatically illustrates the dangers and challenges that patients like this face and that hospital staffs have in treating them.

Come to think of it, he never did say "thank you."

Can't Feel the Burn

Some things physically happen to you that render your appearance different from normal humans. This happens to patients who are victims of burns. The burns of patients who actually qualify to be transferred to the burn unit instead of being treated in the emergency room are of such a high severity that their life and limbs are invariably at imminent risk. This makes every interaction highly intense—and that's not even considering the horror that resides within the patient who survived the episode.

During my first experience working in a burn unit, I distinctly remember a burn patient who came directly to the unit, which isn't the norm. He had substantial full-thickness (third-degree) burns, meaning the burn was so deep that it involved the nerves to an extent that the patient wasn't even in pain. Even worse in the short term, the burn was severe enough that it encased his entire chest. The result of this was that the area had become leathery and constricted as if under a vise grip. In the example of a chest burn, that means a serious restriction of breathing ability and decreased ability to deliver oxygen to the rest of the body. This represents a life-threatening consideration that can lead to diminished healing, heart attacks, and strokes.

My first thought was honestly, *Wow, that kind of looks like E.T.'s chest.* Then, as I pivoted back to being a physician and noticed that this patient was unstable due to the decreasing ability to oxygenate, my immediate next thought was *What exactly am I supposed to do with this?* Even as I collected my thoughts to remember, a nurse handed me a scalpel.

There's a medical procedure called an *escharotomy* in which you basically cut open the charred skin on all sides and watch the skin pop up like bread out of a toaster. When you're doing this, you don't even give any numbing medicine, because the skin doesn't have any feeling, as the local nerves have been burned through. (It's not quite that barbaric: sedatives and pain medicines are offered as needed.) You also don't have an inordinate amount of time to stress over what you're doing, because when this procedure is indicated, it's usually an emergency. The even more amazing thing is that the patient's condition started improving almost immediately.

Although I was in awe of the power I had discovered in my hands, I remember thinking, *Who was the first guy to try this?*

GTSBOOM

Taking care of major trauma patients is done according to protocols. These protocols are based on several considerations, such as whether you were a victim of blunt or penetrating trauma and the parts of your body involved. This provides a wonderful method of quality control, but I often wondered if it wasn't also the case simply because the victims of trauma sometimes can't talk. On other occasions, when they can, they (and their associates) choose not to be exactly forthcoming with information about what just happened. As a result, instead of wasting time, maybe it's best to just get about the business of taking care of them and ruling out the various life threats that could be present.

Here's an example that I'm certain I have heard over one hundred times. In asking a victim of trauma, "What happened to you?" the response is usually a variation of a simple response: "I was walking down the street minding my own business, and I got the stuff beat out of me (GTSBOOM)"—well, that's almost what they say. There's also "I was just standing around, and a bullet seemed to jump on me." Unfortunately, the victims of trauma often came from or are needing to return to an environment that isn't safe and doesn't reward those who snitch. It's a stunning commentary on one's mentality that these types of considerations could be so prominent on someone's mind while they're in pain, bleeding, and at risk of death.

Aside from the fear factor related to future danger, GTSBOOM patients are often facing clear and present dangers.

These patients may be comatose and actually unable to verbalize anything. In those cases, diagnosing the problems becomes like a scavenger hunt and a race against time before something that's damaged turns horribly wrong and life-threatening.

My best advice is that if you or someone you care for is a victim of trauma, do the right thing and provide the medical team all the information you can. Oh yeah, and be careful walking down the street.

The Drama of Major Trauma: When Your Lung Collapses

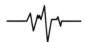

I t's a busy day in a busy trauma center . . .

The squawk box is hot: "We have a twenty-five-year-old male, single gunshot wound to the chest. Vital signs stable. Two minutes out."

Well, that didn't tell much, but they'll be here soon. We're ready.

Preparation is key. Before the patient even arrives, we're set up for many contingencies. In bursts the ambulance. "Doc, he collapsed. He was really having a hard time breathing. We got a (breathing) tube in him."

We get the patient in the trauma resuscitation room. Normally, the paramedics have the patients packaged nicely for us. In this case, there just wasn't enough time. Now, by "collapsed," he meant the patient lost consciousness. Had the patient's heart lost its rhythm, this would be a different process all together.

Airway: No problem there. The paramedics have controlled the airway. Wait. The patient's oxygen level is very low. The tube may not be placed properly . . .

I ask the paramedics: "Is this a good tube? Would you bet his life on it?"

In traumatic arrests, we follow A-B-C, regardless of whatever else is happening, including something obvious and thought to be dangerous, like a knife stuck in his skull. A is for airway. Assessing the airway involves ruling out obstructions or other issues with the airway, which runs from the mouth through the trachea (windpipe) and goes down to the lungs. It is assessed normal by the ability to talk and the presence of a clear and open airway. B is for breathing. Assessing breathing involves checking manifestations of the ability to normally deliver oxygen throughout the body. This includes listening to the various lung fields and noting the absence of the need to use accessory (i.e., backup) muscles to breath. C is for circulation. Assessing circulation involves your blood pressure, which is a measure of the body's ability to distribute blood throughout the body. In any trauma, circulation will be addressed by placing two large-bore IVs to administer fluids and, in some circumstances, blood or blood products.

If there's a problem with A, it must be fixed prior to going to B. The ABCs need to be controlled prior to any other consideration. Back to our patient . . .

Based on the slightest equivocation by the paramedics, the tube is promptly replaced with a larger tube; the larger the tube, the better able we will be to oxygenate the patient. The previous effort may have been good; it doesn't matter. I need 100 percent confidence, as there's a life hanging in the balance. I see my tube pass through the vocal cords. It's in, although it passed with some difficulty. As I listen to the breath sounds (one measure of adequacy of tube placement), I do not hear breath sounds on the side of the gunshot wound. Meanwhile, the patient's oxygen level is low, as is the blood pressure. His heart rate is very fast. I tap on the patient's chest wall and note that the sound is abnormally loud, like the sound produced by the beating of a drum. I look up at the patient's neck, and his trachea (windpipe) is deviated to the left, away from the side of the gunshot wound.

"Get me a 16-gauge needle!"

This patient has a *tension pneumothorax.*

We really take for granted our ability to breathe. There's air everywhere, right? What's the problem? Whatever the problem, consider for a second what it would feel like to have a collapsed lung (pneumothorax). A pneumothorax can either occur spontaneously or, as in this case, it can be the result of some traumatic injury that cuts or punctures the lung. The lung collapses as air escapes from the lung into the space between the lung and the inner portion of your chest wall. With each breath, the amount of air trapped outside of your lung in this space (the *pleural space*) increases, placing additional pressure on your collapsed lung. A *tension pneumothorax* is a life-threatening condition where both respiratory and circulatory collapse has occurred, meaning that the ability to oxygenate and deliver blood through the body is compromised. The patient will die if the situation is not promptly reversed.

I take the large needle the nurse has just given me and ram it (yep, just like a stab) in between two ribs (in the anatomically correct position; please don't try this at home). A large, rapid gush of air is heard, representing release of the trapped air from the pleural space. Almost immediately, the heart rate, blood pressure, and oxygen statuses are normalized, and the trachea has returned to its normal position.

Having avoided this immediate life threat is not the same as saying the patient is out of danger. He is still the victim of a gunshot wound to the chest. However, at this point, airway, breathing, and circulation have been controlled. The needle to the chest will need to be replaced with a much larger chest tube to manage ongoing leakage from the injured lung.

At this point, the trauma surgeon and trauma team have made it to the resuscitation; all of the previous effort actually took about one minute. They will subsequently place the chest tube in, complete the patient's evaluation, and perform any surgery needed (no, this does not include getting the bullet out).

This patient could have died in several different ways in the brief time between when the paramedics got to him and when I completed my handoff to the trauma team. Management of trauma patients is beautiful in its execution, but it is best left undone. You really don't want to have to go through the drama of major trauma.

Caring for Your Friends and Their Families When You Can't Ideally Care for Your Friends and Their Families

I have had three separate occasions wherein, by complete happenstance, friends and/or their family members came to the ER in critical condition when I was on duty. On each occasion, their initial response was the same: "Thank God, YOU'RE here!" On each occasion, my initial response was the same but involved an expletive.

Oddly, in these circumstances, I never happened to be at my normal place of work or in a major emergency department but was working in a smaller community hospital. It certainly isn't true of all community hospitals, but in these examples, my immediate concern wasn't what would happen in the emergency room but what would happen once the patient got admitted to the hospital. I have worked in a lot of places where the skills of the emergency physicians weren't matched by the hospital's ability to provide us with the equipment needed to do our best work. More and more, emergency physicians are made to work around purchasing decisions made not by physicians and without physician input, and in real time, this can pose risks to patients. The irony of this situation is that physicians are made to share the liability for these considerations with the hospital in the event of an adverse outcome to a patient.

These are the thoughts that go through my mind whenever any patient comes in. Hundreds of algorithms race across my brain based on a patient's presenting complaint, including the worst possible scenario. These scenarios are matched with what I know I will need to care for the patient. They are always matched with what I know I will need to do if the appropriate equipment isn't available. All the while, the patient and their families never have a clue about such things. Even as medical directors, physicians have limited, if any, ability to dictate equipment needs to hospitals in the way primary care physicians are able to in their office settings.

In spite of this, I never lost a friend or family member while in my care in an emergency room. However, on more than one occasion, once the patient was stabilized and ready to be transported to the medical floor or Intensive Care Unit, I took the friend aside and advised in the most tactful yet stern way possible that the family member should be transferred elsewhere as soon as possible. In two of those instances, my fears were realized, and the family member died in the hospital. In both of those instances, my friends sought me out to thank me for giving them time to make peace with their loved ones. Yet even to this day, I wonder if things could have turned out differently if they had been able to be transferred to a facility with a higher level of care. I still think of these cases and my affected friends. I hope it's not inappropriate to say I think I'm more affected by what happened than they are.

One of the rules of emergency medicine is that the outcome isn't as important as giving patients the best opportunity to have a good outcome. My ongoing concern is that even when I can personally produce a good outcome, the patient may not be given the best opportunity. I really wish patients had more access and transparency to the inner workings of hospitals.

Time Is Tissue

Consider the following patients:

- A nine-year-old male is brought into the emergency department with sudden onset of pain to the left side of his scrotum. The pain started an hour prior to arrival.
- A twenty-year-old man presents to the emergency department fifteen minutes after a fight. He has a tooth completely knocked out of its socket. He's holding it in his hand.
- A thirty-year-old man presents to the emergency department after sawing off his thumb clean through the joint while at work. He brings it in wrapped in tissue.
- A forty-year-old man presents after his wife has cut off his penis. He has it in a jar soaking in water.
- A fifty-year-old female presents after sudden-onset vision loss in one eye. This occurred twenty minutes prior to arrival.
- A sixty-year-old male with diabetes, hypertension, and a history of smoking presents thirty minutes after the onset of crushing chest pain.
- A seventy-year-old female is brought in by her family after awakening with right-sided weakness, slurred speech, and facial droop.

What all of these patients have in common is they are subject to a very important rule of emergency medicine:

Time Is Tissue.

The entire premise of an emergency department is that there are circumstances in which your cure is rate limited. Even though the overwhelming majority of emergency department patients today are seen for strains and sprains, sniffles and lungs that whistle, moans, groans, and other things that could be cared for at home, every patient we see is being evaluated for a potentially life-threatening condition.

At the time of crisis, the biggest risk patients have is the lack of understanding of what is and isn't important. Although many patients overutilize and inappropriately utilize the emergency room, others fail to come in time to address matters that threaten life and limb. It's understandable, but at some point the inability to have access to the information and advice that can appropriately direct you to the care you need has consequences.

Let's review the cases as examples of this.

The nine-year-old male with groin pain has *testicular torsion*, a twisting of the scrotum, such that the blood supply is interrupted and the scrotum is at risk of dying. The cure rate is up to 100 percent if addressed within six hours of its onset, and there is a very high loss rate if it is unaddressed within eight hours of its onset.

The twenty-year-old man with the tooth knocked out of its socket has ninety to one hundred minutes to get that tooth re-planted. He loses a percentage point of chance of survival of the tooth with every minute the tooth remains out of socket.

The thirty-year-old man with the sawed-off thumb doesn't have a time course for successful replantation, but the longer the thumb is detached, the more likely it is that something else will damage the finger beyond repair.

The forty-year-old with the detached penis has approximately eighteen hours to have it replanted. I will refrain from additional comment.

The fifty-year-old with sudden vision loss has a condition known as *central retinal artery occlusion*. This condition usually results from a clot blocking the blood supply to the eye. This must be treated within ninety minutes of onset to prevent permanent vision loss.

The sixty-year-old male is having a heart attack. His absolute best chances for recovery exist if he gets to the appropriate care setting within ninety minutes of symptom onset.

The seventy-year-old female has had a stroke. Her absolute best chances for recovery exist if she gets to the approximate care setting within three hours of the onset of symptoms. This situation is especially complicated because it may be impossible to know when symptoms started, since they were discovered upon awakening.

If the point you got from these vignettes is that time is important for selected diseases, you have learned only half of what you needed to learn. It should stand to reason that most diseases, whether a skin infection, pneumonia, strep throat, or even an ankle sprain, will get worse with time if you don't learn and take the steps necessary to prevent complications and advancement of disease entities. It starts with acquiring or having access to the knowledge you need when you need it most. Get yours. Your clock may be ticking.

At the Time of Death

An ambulance brings in a patient in cardiac arrest. The patient, a sixty-year-old male with diabetes, kidney failure, and a recent heart attack, collapsed shortly after dinner. He has no spontaneous heartbeat, respirations, or blood pressure. The paramedics have inserted a temporary airway to help deliver oxygen to the patient. They are in the midst of *advanced cardiac life support* (ACLS) and have intermittently elicited an unstable heart rhythm, but it goes in and out. The patient presents twenty minutes after the initial collapse and after eight minutes of the paramedics working on him and transporting him to the emergency department.

When I first started practicing, whenever a patient was in cardiac arrest, the family would stay huddled in the waiting room or family room. They didn't know what was going on, and, honestly, most didn't care to know. I would most often hear, "Do whatever you think is best, doctor."

How times have changed. Families are now encouraged to participate in resuscitation decisions. In many instances, prior to being asked to make decisions about whether or not to continue, patients' families are brought back to see the situation as it exists. In other instances, hospitals encourage families to actually witness the resuscitations if they have the inclination to do so.

What changed? Why would this change be a good thing?

I hear you out there. I'm glad you thought to ask. There are many reasons why this change is for the better.

In the midst of a resuscitation, traditionally, physicians deal with two opposing considerations. On the one hand, we deal with wanting to give patients the best opportunity to come through a likely tragic event. We have the knowledge and technology to continue resuscitative efforts close to indefinitely. We have all seen miracles and know that as long as some chance exists, success is possible. We want you and your loved ones to have that chance.

On the other hand, we understand the notion of medical futility. We are sensitive to the notion of death with dignity. We respect that you may not want your loved one's last experiences to be violent, painful, and traumatic, filled with needles and tubes. (This is why we so strenuously advocate advance directives; they allow your wishes to be communicated before tragedy strikes.)

An additional consideration that I'm pleased to say has gained increasing importance in this equation is the empowerment of a patient's loved ones. Your lasting memories and the way you will be made to live the rest of your lives relative to what occurred during the (potential) death of your loved one are important considerations. Traditionally, you may not have been given the chance to say goodbye or to weigh in on the decision to continue or halt resuscitative efforts. We now know that isn't the healthy position for someone to be in psychologically. Engaging families in the decision, explaining options, and allowing them to come to grips with the choice the physician is pointing them in (or not) leads to a more satisfactory outcome in the long run.

Regarding the patient: I have probably seen that same patient a hundred times with every conceivable outcome. What I can say with certainty is that whether or not these patients have died with dignity or made a miraculous recovery, I want the family to feel the same about the process. We can't guarantee outcomes, but we should be able to guarantee dignity, respect, inclusion, and the best opportunity possible. When the time comes that you're facing this with your family, push to receive the same considerations. You have a voice, and it deserves to be heard.

Working Yourself to Death

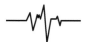

When you have a job, your first priority typically is doing a good job. Safety considerations rarely prevent you from doing your job, although doing your job often prevents you from being safe. Healthcare workers are in constant concern about being exposed to hepatitis and HIV from needle sticks and a multitude of infectious diseases obtained simply by breathing the same air as their patients. Construction workers face the challenges of dust, asbestos, and physical injury. Police officers wonder daily if they may receive a bullet in the line of duty. Firefighters cope with possible burns as well as cyanide and carbon monoxide exposure. And on and on.

There are many workers who spend their entire day outdoors. That makes for a pleasant experience on a beautiful day but can make for a series of life-threatening challenges. Working on a day in which the temperature was over one hundred degrees and the humidity appeared to be just as bad, the emergency department seemed to have turned into a heat exhaustion clinic. Then we were confronted with the challenge we knew all too well would be coming at some point in time.

At about 4:00 p.m., a fifty-year-old, obese male was brought in after collapsing. He was a lineman and had spent the day going up and down poles while wearing relatively heavy protective equipment. Earlier in the day, he had commented to a coworker that he felt like he had been working out all day. He had become increasingly tired and dizzy. Fortunately, he was able to make it down a pole before passing out, where his partner was able to drive him to the emergency department.

The patient was overweight. His skin was quite hot and sweaty. His temperature was over 104 degrees. He was solemn, confused, and speaking slowly. His heart was pounding and racing.

This is a life-threatening emergency.

My staff attacked him, getting him out of his clothes and starting IV fluids in both arms. Measures to get him cooled off as rapidly as possible were taken. We pulled out massive fans and aimed them at him. He was being sprayed with cool water. He had ice packs placed on his groin, armpits, and either side of his neck. We were in a race against the clock. He hadn't had any seizures yet, and I didn't want any to start.

If all of this seems like a bit much, it shouldn't. Heat illnesses actually happen quite often. In fact, they are just as expected in the summer as colds and the flu are in the winter, depending on where you live. Heat illnesses range from heat cramps and heat exhaustion to heat stroke, which is what it appears this patient has. The fact that stroke is in the name should tell you how serious a condition this is. This patient is at risk of several different organs failing and has lost control of his ability to regulate his temperature. He has already demonstrated evidence of damage to his brain by losing consciousness and maintaining some degree of altered mental status. The fact that he is still sweaty is particularly interesting, because in heat stroke, you're usually hot and dry, unless you're suffering from exertional heat stroke (which he could be) or you're obese (which he is). Sweating is an attempt by the body to cool itself, so this could indicate the body still is trying to fight back.

The next step in treating this patient is to quantify the degree of damage. Of particular interest is an evaluation of his liver and kidneys. If either (and especially if both) organ shuts down, the risk to his life increases even more.

Time to take a look at his Foley catheter . . .

A routine procedure in management of ill patients is the placement of a rubber tube into the bladder through the penis or urethra. Draining the bladder accomplishes several goals and tasks. As a waste product, urine is an illustration of what's going on inside of you.

> His urine is cola-colored. Now I need to worry about rhabdo.

A particularly dangerous complication of heat stroke is *rhabdomyolyis* (a.k.a., rhabdo). This is the breakdown of muscle tissue. This breakdown releases muscle fibers into the blood, where they can cause damage to the kidneys, including outright kidney failure. Heat stroke is a particular risk for the development of rhabdo, and the presence of brownish, reddish, or cola-colored urine is a sign that increases suspicion. Blood tests confirm the diagnosis, but no emergency physician is waiting for that before starting treatment. When severe enough, potassium levels increase and threaten the heart, and dialysis may even become necessary.

This patient with heat stroke ends up with damage to his brain and kidneys. We were able to reverse the tide and get his temperature down relatively quickly before even more complications set in. He required a multiple-day stay in the Intensive Care Unit with an eventual recovery.

Patients spend way too much time in the moment of any given illness and oblivious to the danger they may be facing. It doesn't seem unreasonable to expect you to just think through how to protect yourself, especially when it comes to common and frequent activities you engage in. At work, it should be even easier. You're a welder? Wear your goggles. You work in insect control? Wear your protective gear and a mask. You work outdoors? Hydrate early and often. In these extreme circumstances, it can be said that if you're not urinating, you're not drinking enough fluids.

When it comes to what we see in the emergency department, it's true that common things happen commonly. It's also true that our medical conditions are most often traceable and are the consequences of our actions. That's not the same as saying illness is your fault, but your health is your responsibility. Empower yourself with knowledge on simple steps you can take to prevent big medical problems from occurring.

"Crike"

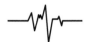

That's medical shorthand for a procedure that is better the less often it needs to be done. It's also an example of how, sometimes, you have to completely think about what you're doing without thinking about what you're doing. If that doesn't make sense to you now, it will by the end of this story.

It's a relatively frequent occasion when a patient needs to be *intubated*. This refers to the process of securing one's airway by placing a breathing tube through the mouth, between the vocal cords, and into the trachea (windpipe). Further down the airway, the trachea branches off several times until branches become components of the two lungs.

Sometimes patients need to be intubated to protect their airways. Examples of this include when one's gag reflex is lost and he or she is vomiting uncontrollably, or when someone is comatose and can't maneuver his or her head and body to control secretions. The latter example seems to occur a lot with various drug ingestions and is especially important because these fluid substances can "go down the wrong tube" (the *esophagus*—feeding tube—is located directly behind your *trachea*—breathing tube). You need to breathe air, not food. Patients also need to be intubated when they have respiratory diseases and are in the midst of an especially bad flare-up. This may occur in asthmatics or those with *COPD* (chronic bronchitis or emphysema). There are still other examples in which unrelated diseases or circumstances affect the patient's respiratory system and ability to oxygenate. Intubation is needed in this case to maintain delivery of enough oxygen to the brain, heart, and other tissues so that you won't have a heart attack or a stroke, among other potential problems.

Intubation itself isn't as bad as it seems (unless you're the patient, I suppose), yet it creates so much angst among the staff and, especially, the families. The families I understand. Intubation involves the use of sedatives and agents to paralyze you—you wouldn't want to be aware of your surroundings with a tube down your throat—and what's more, it's probably the closest your loved one will come to appearing deceased until that time actually comes. I think the staff is just anxious because they know what happens next if the attempts to intubate aren't successful.

A *cricothyrotomy* ("crike" for short) is a medical procedure that, if you saw it, you would swear the physician was slitting someone's throat. It's done when the airway can't be secured (i.e., intubated) through the mouth, either from failed attempts or technical difficulties such as something obstructing the airway, like a peanut or a toy. The decision to perform and the execution of a cricothyrotomy need to be done quickly, such as after three failed attempts at intubation or within ninety seconds, because the risk of the brain and heart suffering increases exponentially.

I have probably successfully intubated a thousand patients. I have had to perform only one cricothyrotomy in my twenty-plus years of practice.

It's a very busy day in a community emergency room; a relatively young male patient comes in wheezing. *Hmm . . . seems like a new onset asthmatic.* Of course, all that wheezes isn't asthma, but the patient is relatively stable even though he does seem to be working kind of hard to breathe. I will briefly talk to and examine the patient and get some things started, but I won't linger. I'm kind of busy because I'm about to deliver a baby in the next room (that's another story).

Well, no more than five seconds after delivering this baby, I hear a piercing scream: "Dr. Sterling!" Nurses are interesting that way. The good, experienced ones are usually so cool, so much so that when they get excited, it's a pretty good clue that something bad just happened.

My would-be asthmatic has collapsed. He is having an extremely hard time breathing and is gasping and using his backup muscles in his chest and abdomen to help himself breathe.

OK . . . not a problem. Let's just "put him down." My nurses gather the medication, and we prepare for what's called a *rapid sequence intubation.* This process gets those sedatives and paralytics (that I discussed earlier) in the patient's system, and they stabilize the patient for the time frame during and after the intubation.

If you're a critical thinker, you may have identified a potential issue: What happens if you paralyze a patient (which includes paralysis of the breathing muscles), and you don't get the breathing tube on board? This challenge is present every time you move to intubate a patient using paralytics. There are both intermittent and definitive options available depending on how critical the situation is.

The patient is ready to be intubated. I have my respiratory therapist on my right and my main nurse on my left. *Let's get this done.* I open the mouth. Insert the blade (the medical device that maneuvers the tongue out of the way). Lift up the palate (the upper inner portion of the mouth) to gain visualization of the vocal cords. Slip the breathing tube between the cords . . . *Hmm . . . it's not passing. That's not right. That's not right . . .*

I regroup and ask for a slightly smaller tube. Open. Lift. Insert. It doesn't pass. *OK. I don't miss . . .* "Give me the crike kit!" I didn't realize gasps made sounds until then. I never did ask my team if they were all gasping because it had just got real or because I had been rendered human. Didn't matter. I had work to do.

Emergency medicine is an especially interesting specialty in that it requires both mental acuity and significant technical expertise. When you're performing a medical or surgical procedure emergently, failure is not an option. Typically, in a small, community hospital, you're the expert, and if you can't do it, it's not going to get done. That's very empowering, because once you accept that, you're done with doubts that want to creep in.

The cricothyroidotomy involves an incision into an area of the throat near the Adam's apple. It's prudent to examine the neck as you're making preparations. I was especially interested in this patient's neck because I was suspicious about what had prevented me from passing the tube down the throat. The patient had denied getting anything stuck in it, but the upper portion of the neck did appear to be protruding . . .

Hmm . . . to the task at hand. That won't affect my procedure. Patient is still sedated and paralyzed. Area is cleaned. I have to identify the area and the membrane I need to puncture. Palm against the chin. I slide my index finger down and back up the throat until I'm in the correct position. *Gain control of the windpipe with one hand. Let's go. Stab incision with only the tip of the scalpel through the membrane, then it's expanded to give me enough room to place the tube. Control the opening with an additional tool and get the tube in there.* We're done in less than twenty seconds. I look up at the nurse. She nods approvingly. I look at the monitor. The oxygen levels are normalizing. I look at the door. Other physicians have come to take the patient to the Intensive Care Unit. I'm done.

No time to rest. I have a baby and newborn mother to check on and an emergency room filled with other patients.

In case you were wondering, the patient had throat cancer that was obstructing the upper airway. The "wheezing" was just the sound of air pushing past the obstructing tumor.

Cutting a Child

Into the emergency department came an eight-year-old child. If the opportunity presents, I'm already evaluating my patients well before I see them in their rooms. It appeared the child's mother was sizing us up as well. This kid was sick. He was pale with a stuttered step. He had one hand over his barf bag (which was covering his mouth) and the other hand covering his belly. It looked like every step he took was painful. The mother's look was not fearful but stern, as if she had switched into Tiger Mom mode. She was here to protect her son. She and I locked eyes. *Let's do this.*

The child had a fever, was vomiting, and had belly pain. The pain was concerning to the mother because it had migrated from the top of the belly down to the bottom, over to the right side. I intentionally shook the bed. As the child jumped up and cried out in pain, his mother jumped up from her chair as if she wanted to beat me up. I held up my hand.

> Ma'am, it appears that your son has a very high probability of having appendicitis.

Her demeanor changed completely. Now, I was her partner.

> Oh my God! What does that mean?

> It means he's going to need surgery.

Then her eyes began to well up with tears.

But he's only eight . . .

This is a very understated consideration. Physicians, particularly emergency physicians, are all about getting down to business. We diagnose the condition, initiate the treatment, and move on to the next patient. We're so inundated with patients that we can easily forget to have human moments. This works well as a self-protective defense mechanism but not so much as a human relating to another human in need.

Appendicitis is the most common surgical emergency in children. It is inflammation of the appendix, which is a small, unneeded, tube-shaped tissue extension off the large intestine. Because it's part of the intestine, it is likely to have stool accumulate inside of it. If it twists off, becomes inflamed, and ruptures, that stool can become expelled into the abdominal cavity. Stool in the abdominal cavity causes an infection that you don't want to have and is life-threatening. Appendicitis was such a concern a few decades ago that surgeons would take many kids to the operating room just to rule out the disease. The prevailing thought of surgeons was that if you had fewer than 20 percent of your patients who didn't have appendicitis discovered during the operation, you weren't operating enough. Surgeons are much more conservative and precise now, partially because it's a child, and it's surgery, after all.

Maybe it was the change in the mother's demeanor that brought the reality of the moment home. Yes, we needed to get that appendix out before it ruptured. Yes, our surgeons were skilled, and this was a routine surgery, but a child was about to get sliced open. Now, physicians don't think of surgery that way, but maybe that was what the mother was thinking.

It suddenly occurs to me that this is like the wheels of a railroad car. On the one hand, all around me, things are happening in a blur. Nurses are rushing to get his blood drawn, an IV started, medicine administered for the nausea and pain, consents signed, a CT scan done, and the surgeon on the phone. That would be the part of the wheel that rotates fast. The mom, the kid, and I are the slower portion. We're sitting there talking about what an appendix is, how appendicitis develops, what the risks are, and why surgery is necessary.

Sometimes all that is heard is "Your child needs surgery." Today, more was heard. They got it. They knew the risks and knew this gave him the best chance to be OK. Once Mom reached up to give me a hug, I figured that was her way of telling me thank you—both for taking care of him and of her. The child would end up fine.

Say My Name!
Screaming Nurses

I love nurses. Always have. Always will. Nursing has always prided itself on being "the caring profession," and knowing the things they are made to do for patients, that is certainly true. The amount of humility and compassion it takes to perform their job is substantial. Nurses also care for doctors (especially the ones they like!), and the smart doctors take care of their nurses at every opportunity. I became a much better physician once I learned to trust and listen to my nurses. Even when they're wrong or off-base about the specifics of a case, they are usually right about something significant being in play. The vast majority of nurses I have worked with clinically are true professionals. They are interested in patient care and are devoted to making me and my medical practice successful. They have allowed me to teach them and show them how to recognize danger signs and things I have expressed that could be important. That helps them communicate things back to me.

In general, my nurses end up with very similar traits. They ask questions and make suggestions. They know when it's OK to drag me by the collar into a room! And then there is the screaming.

As a physician, you can learn to loathe your name. I'm sure there were days when I heard "Dr. Sterling" over a thousand times. It is always a special treat to have five people conversing with me simultaneously. That said, the nurses always knew how to get my attention.

- There was the "Dr. Sterling," as in "You really aren't paying attention."
- There was the "Dr. Sterling," as in "Stop, and listen to me."
- There was the "Dr. Sterling," as in "Please don't make me do that!"
- There was the "Dr. Sterling," as in "I don't care if you haven't eaten, I have a question."

However, those were the stern voices. There were also the screams.

- "Dr. Sterling"—sing-song, as in "One of your inappropriately flirty patients is here!"
- "Dr. Sterling"—annoyed, as in "Where are you hiding?"
- "Dr. Sterling"—pleading, as in "When are you going to do what I asked you to do? We need to get this patient out of here!"
- "Dr. Sterling"—afraid, as in "Someone's trying to die!"

One day, I heard a scream that I had never heard before, and I'm sad to say I have heard it several times since. The shriek sounded like my nurse was in danger. I rushed to the room and slung open the curtain. There stood my nurse, almost in tears. She was standing there like someone had just thrown a bucket of water on her.

My eyes darted to the patient, a seventy-something-year-old male, laid back on the stretcher. My nurse was engaged in a routine process of placing a *catheter* (drainage tube) into his penis. The patient had an enlarged prostate that was obstructing the flow of urine from his bladder; the catheter would release the urine and any associated pressure and pain.

Apparently, as she grasped his penis and manipulated it to facilitate passage of the catheter, the patient had a rather massive orgasm, which managed to spray on the nurse.

What do you think my response was? Yep, a different type of scream!

You're Gonna Be a
Great Doctor!

In many cases, practicing medicine is filled with subtleties. Anatomical positioning is important when performing procedures, lest complications occur. Checking and rechecking medication doses prevents under- or overdosing. Even something as simple as a physical examination requires a demonstration of expertise.

For example, there is a meaningful difference between massaging and palpating an object. You understand what a massage is. It's a caress meant to relax and impart pleasure. *Palpating* an object communicates back to you various aspects of the object. It's feeling with a medical purpose, meant to examine an object's texture, location, or tenderness. Trust me; this is a distinction with a difference.

As a medical student, once we were finally allowed to get our heads out of our books and onto some real-world activity, one of the first things that was important to learn and master was how to appropriately perform a physical exam. Everything from head to toe, inside and out, needs to be addressed meticulously. You need to know what you're looking for and how to find it. One of the rules of emergency medicine is that lab tests confirm diagnoses, not make them. A good history and physical exam will teach you everything you need to know in most cases.

Interestingly, and to that end, on Fridays the medical students would engage in an activity we called "anatomy massage happy hour." As a means of learning all the muscles, bones, and other structures of the body, we would practice on each other. In retrospect, maybe we should have left out the massage and happy hour portions, or at least replaced the massage with palpation.

I had one of my early student rotations (month-long experiences in different medical settings) in obstetrics and gynecology at a Planned Parenthood facility. I would imagine I was about twenty-three or twenty-four at the time. In any setting, even now as an experienced emergency physician, it's important to have a female attendant with you when performing examinations on females. This works for your safety as well as for the patient's. There have been far too many cases in which patients have been assaulted and otherwise violated for this not to be the case. Similarly, physicians have been accused of performing acts that either didn't occur or didn't occur intentionally.

I am presented with a young, attractive, female patient who comes in for a routine checkup. I am joined by the nurse (who happens to be a nun) for the physical examination. I am pulling out my best bedside manner so as to make the patient comfortable. I'm diligent and focused on what I'm supposed to feel and how everything is supposed to feel. At this stage of my development, everything is deliberate and takes a bit longer than it will eventually.

I get to the pelvic examination last. That begins with an external examination. I'm entirely inside of my head at this point, but I'm very careful to explain everything that's occurring as I go along.

OK. Normal-appearing female genitalia. No rashes, lesions, or ulcers. Nothing seems especially tender or uncomfortable.

I progress to the speculum exam. *OK; let's make sure the speculum is warm and appropriately sized. She has a normal-appearing cervix. No discharge or lesions noted. Let's get these specimens done.*

Now to the bimanual exam. *Everything is good. The uterus (womb) is not enlarged or tender. I don't feel any abnormalities up by the ovaries. The cervix is long, thick, closed, and non-tender.*

I had completely forgotten that I was examining a person, even though I was speaking to her the entire time. When I finished, I took off the gloves I had been using and prepared to do a breast examination. I looked up at the patient, and she was flushed and smiling.

You're going to be a grrrreat doctor!

I look at the nun nurse, who is beet red. I immediately walk out of the room, not to return. *Mental note to self: There's a difference between feeling and palpating. You need to practice.*

Oh, the Horror

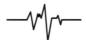

A young, first-time mother bursts into the emergency room in the middle of the night, sobbing uncontrollably. She's holding her two-year-old son in her arms. He appears to be in no acute distress.

> My baby! How did this happen? Please . . . help him.

> Sure, we're happy to help. What brings you in to see us?

> I was checking on him. I thought I smelled a wet diaper, so I checked it. And . . . then . . . I saw worms down there! It was horrible! Is my baby going to be OK?

> Yes. If it's what I think it is, he should be OK. Let's take a look.

First-time mothers are unique. It can be very hard to convince some that you're actually on their side. They can be nervous, afraid, and very suspicious; if the physician is not successful in establishing the right bond and instilling confidence in these mothers that he or she is interested and taking them seriously, they will take offense. They may not always understand fully what's wrong, but when they "know" something is wrong and you haven't addressed the concern to their satisfaction, it's very difficult to console them without appearing uncaring. In some cases, even after you have explained the problem, the fear doesn't dissipate.

I never want to be wrong when taking care of a baby, but in this case, you feel as if you're caring for both mother and child. You just know these mothers would never forgive themselves for trusting anyone if something bad happened to their children. No mother wants to live to see the death of her child, and if it happened in a hospital, that would be unacceptable. Thus, even if the presentation is something routine, it is very important to discuss the full range of possibilities, because the mother is especially fearful of this being the tip of the iceberg.

Pinworms are a huge advertisement for the value of hand washing and keeping your hands off of your face. Microscopic pinworm eggs are found on surfaces such as bed linens, towels, clothes, toys, toilets, and feeding utensils. They get digested and migrate to the large intestines and around the rectum, where they live as parasites and cause itching. Children who scratch the itch can reintroduce the cycle by placing their hands (containing new eggs) back in their mouths. The most frequent time to see the worms is a few hours after the child has gone to sleep. The worms may also be seen in the toilet or in the child's underwear.

All of this is explained to the mother, whose expression never changes from sheer horror. "Does this mean he'll be deformed? Will he grow?" I'm doing my best, but the ultimate question always follows: "Are you sure?" *I sure hope so. Well, that's what I'm thinking, but she needs a definitive yes.*

I explain the "cellophane tape test" to her, which is redundant at this point but empowers her. This test involves Mom taking a piece of clear cellophane tape and applying it near the anus. This is likely to provide definitive evidence, as the worms will get stuck on the tape when they emerge. In the meantime, we can treat the child with one dose, and if symptoms recur, we will treat the entire family.

She appears satisfied, and I'm relieved. I ask her if I can do anything else just as often as she asks me, "Are you sure?" This is important work, even if it's frustrating. That goes for both of us, but on this occasion, I think we both got it done. No job is too small when it comes to caring for a patient in the ER. One of the rules of emergency medicine is that *perception is reality*, and the way that rule applies here is until Mom is satisfied, we really haven't done our best work.

Just Get on the Bed and Yank!

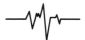

Part of the aura physicians have involves a veil of professionalism. Even as we joke with you, we're always mindful of our need to be "professional." It's hard sometimes. We're not a bunch of robots walking around without feelings, emotions, or senses. We smell the odors you know are there. We see what you have done. We hear what you just said. Sometimes you make us want to laugh, cry, scream, and just release it all. Instead, we master the art of "umm hmm."

We also are put into positions where what we're doing is either so silly or incredible that you deserve to laugh at us, or at least, we should be willing to laugh at ourselves. Many times, what's most funny about what we're doing is trying to remain professional in the face of something completely absurd.

I had a patient who was somewhat famous in his community. He was a big, strong guy who was known to tie one over at the bars and get into brawls. It seemed like this happened every Friday night. The locals, finally tired of being on the losing end of bar fights, devised a strategy. It appears the big, strong guy had a weakness. He had a problem with hip dislocations. His right hip was known to pop out of its socket from time to time. Their strategy was to kick him on the front side of his upper thigh and pop his femur (the thigh bone reaching into the hip joint) out of place. Then the group would pile on him until he gave in. This was a very cruel strategy. Hip dislocations are incredibly painful, and you cannot move with your femur out of socket.

I saw this patient on multiple occasions and was always impressed that nothing more serious was wrong with him. Even after a full evaluation, it always came down to getting his femur back in place and allowing him to sober up.

About that hip . . . Hip dislocations are interesting. The hip generally is incredibly stable. The head of the femur is shaped like a ball and fits snugly into the hip joint. It really takes a lot to get it out. It also takes a lot to get it back in.

Thinking back to my training as an emergency physician, everything was so precise and meticulous. The best way to perform a procedure is to prepare and set the conditions for success. The technique never fails if appropriately applied with anatomic precision. In the case of a reduction of a dislocated hip, that means you give a lot of muscle relaxers and pain medication. You have someone hold the hips down while you stabilize the foot against your thigh, bend the knee, and lift the knee toward the sky (don't try this at home). This procedure never fails—until it does.

When you're in specialty training, you often think of the adage "do no harm." Hip dislocations are often associated with fractures and have a high complication rate. The reduction of a dislocation can present its own challenges and complications, so until you become familiar with the procedure, you tend to be less definitive and more gentle. On those occasions that the previous approach to the procedure wouldn't work, I recalled the voice of one of my supervising physicians during my training, yelling at me: "Just get on the bed and yank!"

So, on the more difficult cases, I would find myself standing on the stretcher with the patient's leg across my shoulder. While someone was holding the hips down, I would basically be doing the equivalent of squats. Once you elicited a pop that could be heard across the room, the femur was back in the socket. I can only imagine how silly I looked in my shirt, tie, and lab coat standing on a bed and squatting in front of this patient's crotch.

Every physician in our local emergency medicine group got a few turns putting this patient's femur back in place. I believe I saw him three to five times. No matter how much I counseled him, he would find his way back on a Friday night. Then, just like that, he disappeared, and I never saw or heard from him again. I wonder if the locals did anything to him . . .

When Someone Tells You
They Are about to Die

When you're a young, impressionable physician, you learn lessons from everything. Medicine is a big mystery, involving science, psychology, and spirituality. Throughout their careers, most physicians would admit to having seen things that were entirely predictable, as well as other things that were completely beyond explanation based on anything learned in medical school. Sometimes this works out well, but other times, what occurs is exactly what you hoped to never have happen.

I remember being brought into a room with a young adult patient who was so anxious and hyperactive that she had been strapped to the bed with leather restraints. She was in the midst of a condition known as *thyroid storm*, which is an extreme, life-threatening case of a hyperactive thyroid. This typically occurs due to hyperthyroidism being untreated, combined with a simultaneous stress such as an infection. Symptoms are dramatic and include agitation, altered mental status, diarrhea, fever and sweating, shaking and tremors, and pounding and rapid heartbeats. In other words, your entire body is malfunctioning, you know it, you can't control it, and it's overwhelming you physically and mentally.

I walked into the room, and she sat up as straight as she could, given the restraints. She looked me right in the eye and said, "I'm about to die!" My first thought was to check and see if she was on cocaine or PCP, but reviewing her history allowed me to figure out pretty rapidly what was actually occurring.

It then occurred to me that I had never heard anyone say that to me. Given that I had never actually managed a case of thyroid storm (even though I knew exactly how to), I knew that with this particular diagnosis—unlike many others—it didn't matter as much if you did everything properly. The risk of death actually was there and would continue to be, simply as a function of the disease being present.

Before long, I had both a thyroid specialist (an *endocrinologist*) and our Intensive Care Unit specialist with me, and we were all managing the patient together. There was a lot of watching and waiting. It had taken her a while to get into this situation, and it would take a while to get her out of it. There are multiple medications needed to treat thyroid storm, but they need to be given in a specific order, and in total, they take over an hour to administer.

What stays with me about this case is how transfixed I was. It is extremely rare in a busy emergency that you stay with one patient for an indefinite period of time. For one of the few times that I can recall, even though I stayed in the room and mostly in the same spot, I avoided eye contact with this patient as much as I could, even as I knew she never took her eyes off of me. I recall standing for almost an hour waiting and treating and looking at the heart and lung monitors and examining and waiting.

I was told once that the problem with thyroid storm is that it is akin to running one hundred miles an hour while on fire. You could slow down gradually, but you're likely to keep burning while you're trying to slow down. You could stop by running into a brick wall, but, of course, you have run into a brick wall and might explode. What you're really hoping for is for the fire to burn itself out. Unfortunately, complications of thyroid storm involve the lungs flooding with fluid, a severe case of congestive heart failure known as *pulmonary edema*. If you're breathing fluid instead of air and this is occurring on top of the thyroid storm, at some point, your body isn't going to be able to fight all of these fights.

The last time she and I made eye contact was before she was about to be sedated in order to allow us to place her on a breathing apparatus (i.e., intubate her). I still can't reconcile what the last look she gave me meant. I think it was less of a "help me" than a "let me go." She wasn't crying but was clearly in agony from the condition that had snatched her body's functions from her.

I have had two other instances in which patients told me with complete certainty that they were going to die on that day. Both were calm, resigned to their perceived fate, and later died after being admitted to the hospital. They both had substantial enough disease that they could have been right or wrong. On the other hand, I have never had a patient tell me they were about to die and be wrong. Of course, that doesn't stop you from doing your best to prevent that fate. It just makes you wonder, and it certainly makes you realize that perhaps the job is more to give patients the best possible opportunity to get better and to facilitate God's will and whatever comes next than to be deluded and filled with God complexes.

The Great,
Grateful Deadheads

Happiness is such a subjective thing. Practicing medicine has brought me a lot of joy over the years. It's not just the lives saved or changed. It's the people. There are so many different types of people living so many different types of lives; being exposed to them is a study in human nature and all that it involves. Emergency medicine has its share of drama and trauma. That is baked in the proverbial cake. The moments of joy held within the drama of the emergency room are special opportunities to view firsthand how all parts of "the other half" live. Sometimes it's the birth of a baby. Other times it's reversing a previous diagnosis of cancer and discovering it was something much less severe. No matter what the medical concern, there are people and moments that embody joy and happiness that are infectious in themselves.

For decades, fans of the rock band the Grateful Dead have traveled around the country with the band. Every summer, the band would roll into town for an extended stay. During the time they were in town, two occurrences would become more prominent around the emergency room: the presence of tie-dye shirts and mushroom intoxication.

Early symptoms of mushroom intoxication and poisoning are fairly nonspecific and include nausea, vomiting, diarrhea, abdominal pain, fatigue, dizziness, and headache. Of course, there are also the hallucinations and euphoria that serve as the incentives for the ingestions. Many other symptoms may become part of the complex as toxicity increases. Serious mushroom poisoning can be life-threatening and most notably involves liver failure. However, the presence of these patients, who would fill up the emergency rooms across the city, wasn't an entirely negative experience for either the patients or the emergency room staff.

I recall a saying I would hear from time to time: Deadheads are high whether or not on drugs. Back then my immediate thought was *Good, so stop doing the darned mushrooms.* In time, I came to realize that this mentality was part of their lives. They traveled, partied, engaged in fellowship, and sometimes got sick. The occasional person would actually die. I didn't have a single unpleasant episode with any of them, even though some would be vomiting their brains out (figuratively, of course) and some ended up critically ill. This certainly isn't an endorsement of any illicit behavior, but it is an effort to make a fair observation. I imagined this wasn't much different than the college-aged students who'd travel to Europe or some other destination for the summer or than the "love, peace, and soul" caravans prominent back in the 60s.

I must admit that it was easy to get caught up in the spirit of it all. When the band would roll out of town and the tie-dye disappeared, you couldn't help but notice the smiles weren't as ubiquitous. On the other hand, there wasn't as much vomiting and diarrhea, either.

When Chicken Pox Kills

I had never heard of such a thing.

I'm working in our emergency department and in comes a frail, female patient in her thirties. She looks toxic and has a high fever, appears fatigued, and has a diffuse rash that looks a lot like chickenpox. However, she's already had chickenpox before as a child.

> Hmm . . . I have heard this was possible but have actually never seen it.

As it turns out, this patient also has HIV/AIDS. That explains a lot. Patients who have diminished immune systems are susceptible to organisms that otherwise might not cause disease even if infected by them. Even worse, organisms that infect patients with lowered immunity are much more dangerous and deadly.

In the emergency department, we start special antiviral antibiotics, provide supportive treatment, and get her admitted to the hospital. I thought that was the end of it.

As luck would have it, I had occasion to work on the medical floors two months later. The patient still has not left the hospital. She is increasingly sick, and infectious disease specialists are primarily managing her at this point. She is located on a unit designed for both contact and respiratory isolation. She is going to die soon.

Is she dying from HIV/AIDS or varicella zoster *(the organism that causes chickenpox)?*

I didn't know if that was a distinction without a difference at the time, but the fact of the matter is that the patient had developed a pneumonia caused by varicella zoster. The HIV/AIDS set the table for her infection, but, in fact, the infection that ended up taking her life was the same one that caused her chickenpox.

What illnesses could have been communicated from her? Why was she in both respiratory and contact isolation?

Pneumonia is a respiratory disease. The respiratory pathogen could have been disseminated through the air, but in an individual with normal immunity, developing an infection similar to that which this patient had wouldn't have been expected. The even more interesting question involves the patient's blisters. They would have been expected to contain chickenpox, but in an HIV/AIDS patient, the HIV virus likely was also in the fluid contained within the blisters. Under certain circumstances, this could have served as a source of transmitting the disease.

This patient was in absolute agony every time I saw her, and I don't mean the type of routine pain and suffering unfortunately seen during the end stages of many diseases. I believe her to have suffered as much and for as long of a time as any patient I have seen in my career. It was painful for her to breathe, to move, and to simply exist.

It's obvious that a certain cautionary tale exists here, but the other thought that burns in my memory is that for some patients, hospice care isn't sufficient and euthanasia isn't an option. This patient had no way to escape a half-living hell for the last two months of her life. It was such a shame that no option existed to deal with her reality.

Did You Get the Bullet Out?

The circumstance doesn't matter.

- Gunshot wound to the head . . . The patient is in a coma.
- Gunshot wound to the chest . . . The patient is on life support.
- Gunshot wound to the back . . . The patient is paralyzed.
- Gunshot wound to the belly . . . The patient is receiving blood and heading to surgery.

After a trauma involving a gunshot wound, right after "Did he make it?" and "Is he going to be OK?" is that question. It gets asked anew by every person who comes to visit.

I don't understand the obsession with bullets. It's as if somewhere along the line someone decided that if a bullet were left in too long, it would start to back up and ricochet around your body like the ball does in a pinball game. On the other hand, some individuals will reveal soon after telling you their name that they have a bullet in them, as if it's a badge of honor—and, of course, many songs actually do reference retained bullets in the context of being a badge of honor and references about being "bulletproof."

Basically, when you come in as the recipient of a gunshot wound, at the beginning of the process, the importance of the bullet is not in the bullet itself but in the damage done by the bullet. There will be any number of things more important in the initial management of a trauma patient than the location of the bullet.

Subsequently, once higher, life-saving priorities have been successfully addressed and the location of the bullet has been identified, the next item of relevance related to the bullet is whether or not it's in a position that will continue to cause damage if left in. If this is the case, a decision may be made to go after it, but that's entirely based on a risk-benefit analysis by your surgeon.

Beyond those considerations, if the bullet is located in an extremely accessible location where no damage will be done by taking it out (as a convenience), the surgeon or emergency physician may decide to do so.

Other than these considerations, will we get the bullet out? No. In most cases, going after the bullet isn't worth the trouble it will cause going after it.

After all, in many cases, when we did get the bullet out, it ended up being placed on a necklace.

When You Do
What You Have To

Every now and again, the police will pick up patients who appear to be in trouble and escort them to the emergency department. This happens a lot during the extremes of weather. This sometimes happens with homeless individuals who appear to be in harm's way. It's interesting when the police choose to do this, as they could conceivably be doing this all the time. Somehow, they know the difference, and, often, their doing so makes a difference.

One afternoon, a patient was brought into the emergency department who was pretty clearly homeless. He was covered in dirt, dressed in layers, and had what appeared to be his personal belongings with him. The concern expressed by the police officer was that he had seen the patient eating dirt and looking disoriented.

In speaking with the patient, he just appeared tired. We spent the next two hours evaluating his baseline medical status and rehydrating him. While talking with him, we discovered he indeed had a habit of ingesting certain non-food substances, including dirt and rocks. Foreign bodies were noted passing through his digestive tract, but not in a way that posed a danger of perforating his stomach or intestines.

Pica is a medical condition that fits this description, but it isn't restricted to the homeless. It's a habit of ingesting non-food substances—not as a mental disorder, but as a result of cravings due to nutritional deficiencies. It is seen disproportionately in younger children and during pregnancy.

Of course, this case is about more than a craving. In this patient, the craving resulted out of necessity and an inability to obtain food in normal ways. With a homeless population estimated at 100 million worldwide and up to 1.75 million in the United States, the scope of pica and many other consequences of homelessness are yet to be discovered.

We hoped the two hours spent in the emergency department were somewhat of a relief for the patient. We fed him and did what we could for the time we had him. On a relative scale, this gentleman was better off than most. Almost two-thirds of the homeless have problems with drug abuse, alcohol abuse, or mental illness. This patient did not appear to have any of these issues, although that was of little comfort. It's unfortunate to say, but it was obvious that some members of the staff were happy to see him leave. That seemed to be a metaphor for much of our approach to homelessness; we would rather they were out of sight.

As is the case with many patients, we are forced to return patients back into the same conditions that produced the pathology in the first place. As he struggled to leave the emergency department, we could only hope that he would be in as good of physical and mental condition if we saw him again.

When the Erection Lasts
More Than Four Hours

You've heard the commercials. They're a bit disingenuous, as many men view the prospect of a four-hour erection as a good thing. If the manufacturers were really interested in creating a deterrent, they would show a commercial displaying what happens next.

Into my busy emergency room comes a studly looking male, aged somewhere in his thirties. He's accompanied by a skittish and clearly freaked-out female. The male would do well to be the one skittish and freaked out. I don't know if his cavalier attitude is due to being oblivious to the situation or to a belief that there is a pill for everything and this situation can easily be addressed. He chose to use an erectile dysfunction pill out of convenience instead of a need, so he could "impress" his girl.

There's not much to say about the examination. He had an erection.

As we sit down to discuss treatment options, you can see his demeanor change. She shakes her head and leaves the room. There are going to be a lot of needles involved.

First, he needs to receive numbing medicine. This is not going to be pretty or pleasant. I'm using the smallest needles we have to anesthetize the area, but he's hopping around the bed like a bunny rabbit going backwards.

We need to get this under control. There is a clear and present danger that needs to be addressed. He is made to understand that the quality of anesthesia is vital for what comes next. I give him a towel to bite on and in which to scream. My nurses are telepathically sending me messages about how men can't tolerate pain. I can hear them in my thoughts as I gaze at one nurse's controlled, bemused smirk. *That's the smallest needle we have. Wonder how he's going to handle the big one.*

Once that's done, I again explain what's about to occur.

We switch from the smallest needle to about the biggest one. The procedure is called *corporal aspiration*. That's medical jargon for I take this needle (attached to a container called a syringe) and insert it into either side of the tissue of his penis (don't try this at home—as if, right?). I then manually extract as much blood as possible (I trust that you do realize that erections are engorgement of the penis with blood, not rigidity of some "bone"). I'm also flushing the area to get rid of any sludged blood. Don't worry; my patient is doing OK. I think he passed out when he first saw the needle.

Despite the drama of this trauma, this drainage procedure works only 30 percent of the time, and my patient is not one of the lucky ones. Next up is insertion (yes, directly into the penis) of a medication that constricts the blood vessels of the penis. This works because it runs against the mechanism of the erection, which is the opening of the blood vessels, allowing the blood to flow to the penis. This procedure actually needed to be repeated three different times, but it got the job done.

Erectile dysfunction is serious business. It affects between fifteen and thirty million men in the US; approximately half of men between forty and seventy deal with some degree of erectile difficulty. The use of newer erectile dysfunction meds has improved the quality of life for many couples. However, their use is not without side effects.

The side effect from which this patient suffered is called *priapism*. Priapism is an unwanted, intractable erection. It really is a medical emergency. Ironically, it can lead to damage of the penis and permanent erectile dysfunction. Just understand that using erectile dysfunction medications for convenience is not without risk.

I don't know who came up with the idea that four hours was an acceptable period of time to maintain a continuous erection, but given the nature of the emergency, I wouldn't wait that long. Think about it. I bet my patient did the next time he had sex.

Extracting Life from Death

Where you choose to live is a very important and personal decision. From a health standpoint, the accessibility of different types of services can make all the difference in the world, whether it's regarding routine care or treatment of life-threatening considerations. It is also a very important decision for the emergency physician to decide where to practice. There's a world of difference between facilities. On the one hand, many physicians practice in a level 1 trauma center, supported by every possible subspecialist with seemingly unlimited equipment and resources within the hospital. At the other extreme, you can find yourself practicing in a remote rural facility where you may be the only available physician for miles. Quality care is wherever you find it, but in my experience, working in different types of facilities has brought unique challenges.

One of the odder cases I recall was a case of a mother who was the victim of a high-speed motor vehicle crash in a remote location on the outskirts of a rural community. Apparently, in attempting to avoid a truck while slipping on dangerous winter roads, she turned her pickup truck head-on into a light pole. She was nine months pregnant; in not wanting to hurt her pregnancy, she had chosen not to wear a seat belt. During the crash, she was propelled over the steering wheel into the windshield. The trucker was courteous enough to stop, check on her, and get help.

Between the time of the accident, arrival of the ambulance, extraction from the vehicle, and transport, approximately fifty minutes had passed. That had to have seemed like an eternity. I shudder to think of the horror everyone involved must have felt. The sad reality was that much of that time was spent trying to resuscitate (i.e., revive) her. She went into cardiac arrest several times during transport, even completely losing her heart rate and rhythm on a few occasions. Significant efforts to save her life were made, but to no avail. The last efforts had been approximately fifteen minutes prior to arrival in the emergency room.

Back at the emergency room, I have known about this evolving situation for approximately fifteen minutes. The sobering reality is, based on what I find, I will have to make a series of horrific decisions. However, first things first: the initial decision is that they need to bring the patient into the emergency room, even though they're ready to pronounce her dead. Additional decisions will involve these considerations:

- There is a mother whose life is at risk and, unbeknownst to me initially, has ended. I have to be prepared to implement advanced cardiac life support in an effort to keep her alive.
- Yes, there is a term pregnancy potentially ready to survive if delivery is needed. That still isn't the first consideration. The best treatment of a fetus is always treatment of the mother. The greatest risk to a fetus is risk to the mother. Pregnancies are well protected inside the mother's belly. Generally, the greater concern is to be found in the fact that fetuses are basically parasites, completely dependant on healthy and functioning mothers.
- Another consideration is what to do if the mother dies. Should you let things go and assume the baby can't survive? Can you figure it out in time? Are there heroic efforts to be made?

It's only a slight exaggeration to say that the time it took to read those last few sentences is about the time one has to choose between those options and make a decision once the patient actually shows up. The real concern is whether an emergency C-section will be necessary.

By the time the ambulance came through the door, they already knew my intentions, so they came in gangbusters, even though the patient was dead. In the time it took to transport the patient to the resuscitation room, there was time for three questions:

- How long has she been in *asystole* (a.k.a., flatlined, without a heartbeat or rhythm)?
- Have you done *CPR* (cardiopulmonary resuscitation) the entire time?
- The third question, which is "What's her gestational age (i.e., how far along is the patient's pregnancy?)," had already been answered by her ob-gyn doctor, who was thirty minutes away and making his way in.

There is a simultaneous amount of horror and hope involved in cutting through a freshly deceased patient's abdomen to save her full-term baby. Technically, it's called an emergency C-section, but in the emergency room, it doesn't resemble any C-section you have ever seen. No matter the need for the procedure, it still feels like a "medically precise slashing." From the time you become aware that the need to do this exists to the time you make the incision, the spectrum of dignity for the dead hovers over you amidst the action you're about to take, which seems to violate that thought. Fortunately, there's no time to reflect on the gravity of the moment; there's only time to act.

You have absolutely no idea what you will find when you extract that baby from inside its mother's womb. If you do know, it's because you took too much time to assess the situation. Survival is directly related to time; in fact, survival is not likely if more than twenty minutes have passed from the time the mother's heart first stopped. Seconds matter here as much as any circumstance in medicine.

In the moment that I cut through the womb and pulled out the fetus, I had a feeling unlike any other in my life. Beyond the horror and hope lie shock and awe. You're simultaneously completely in the moment in the room with the patient and elsewhere in purgatory, where life and death is in the balance.

Many of us, mindful of the sacrifices others have made for us, know the burden of living a life that honors that sacrifice. I can only wonder what that little girl will make of her life.

Sizzurp

I had a patient who would show up to the emergency department about once a week. She was the sweetest, most polite patient. She had been a long-time smoker and now suffered from chronic bronchitis. All she ever wanted was promethazine (the generic name for a common anti-nausea preparation) with codeine, because she coughed so much that she stayed nauseated. The promethazine wasn't a problem, but the codeine was. Emergency departments are rapidly getting out of the business of providing refills on narcotic pain medications to patients. These are medicines meant to be prescribed by a primary care physician. However, in the midst of an emergency, such as an acute exacerbation of bronchitis, one might conceivably offer a short-term amount. Well, this patient had figured this out. The combination of sweet, charming, and sick proved to be such a mixture that just often enough, between as many emergency departments as she was frequenting, she was able to get enough promethazine with codeine to stock a pharmacy.

I had another patient who came in after sawing part of his finger off. Why would he do this, you ask? He was intoxicated, but not by alcohol. While high, he and his friends decided to engage in some woodwork. Believe it or not, he actually fell asleep (well . . . not for long).

A word to the parents. You might want to read this closely. There has been a long tradition of children and teenagers using common household items and over-the-counter medications as a means of getting intoxicated. If you're interested in preventing that from happening, the first item you should secure in your home is alcohol. If you have a bar and you have teenagers, please consider locking up your liquor. Do you remember the joys of sniffing glue? Guess what? Just because it went "out of style" doesn't mean it's not still effective and no longer poses a risk. How often are you checking the level of your glue supply? How about spray paint and other aerosols that can be inhaled using a plastic bag?

The first patient referenced, the sweet, charming, frequent visitor to the emergency department, reminds me of the latest trend in this tradition, to which the second patient fell prey. Purple Drank (a.k.a., sizzurp, Texas tea, and other names) is the result of mixing prescription-strength cough syrup with one of several beverages, such as Big Red, Sprite, or Mountain Dew (a Jolly Rancher candy is often added as well). The promethazine has a purple color, hence the name. This mixture is just sweet enough to appeal to teenagers and young adults.

These substances are simple ways of getting high off of codeine. The promethazine is considered a "doorstop" against an overdose. It has a side effect of drowsiness, so theoretically, one would fall asleep before overdosing on the codeine. That doesn't work. There have been several notable high-profile overdoses in the entertainment industry, including the individuals who popularized the concoction.

There are at least two other flaws in this strategy. It assumes that no one is chugging the drink. Of course, that's not the case, and as a result, several cases of these ingestions present to emergency departments with the appearance of a codeine overdose. The other flaw is that it assumes that you're staying at home and not operating heavy machinery. I have also cared for patients involved in motor vehicle crashes after falling asleep at the wheel due to Purple Drank intoxications, in addition to the finger amputation.

If there's a lesson to be learned here, it's to first be mindful of the items floating around your house. That must be coupled with securing potentially dangerous items. Childproofing your house can't be limited to placing covers on outlets. On the other hand, maybe that's why neighbors are always rummaging through your medicine cabinets.

Flying through the
Intersection of Health
and Happiness

It's a beautiful summer day. You know, the type when you enjoy wearing as little as possible. You would never think about it that way, but that actually increases the risk for some of us.

The ambulance squawk box speaks: "We have a MVC (motor vehicle collision): motorcycle vs. car. Biker ejected. Multiple blunt trauma with LOC (loss of consciousness) for five minutes. He's A&Ox3 (alert and oriented to person, time, and place—that means he still has his mental bearings) and a GCS of 10 (that's an acronym for a coma scale used to follow trends in neurologic functioning—15 would be normal). He has obvious injuries to both arms and legs. We have him on *C-collar* (hard neck brace) and a backboard and have established two large bore IVs. We'll see you in five minutes."

According to the US National Highway Traffic Safety Administration, a motorcyclist's risk of a fatal crash is thirty-five times greater than the driver of an automobile. A study from the Centers for Disease Control and Prevention, covering a seven-year period, estimated that over 1,222,000 persons were treated in US emergency departments for non-fatal motorcycle injuries, with another 34,000 motorcyclists suffering fatal injuries.

The facts and the experiences I have with motorcycle injuries have affected me as dramatically as most things about medicine. When I was completing my emergency medicine training, one fact that stayed with me from the trauma team was that active motorcyclists can expect to have an accident (to a statistical certainty) within five years of biking. What's worse is that the bikes themselves basically provide no protection from injury. What's even worse is the insistence of some individuals to ride motorcycles without helmets or any other protective clothing. What's not understandable is when someone says that's exactly the point and part of the thrill—it's about the freedom. So I don't judge. I just wait to treat.

That logic worked until the patient involved in this accident ended up being everyone's favorite nurse. He was the life of the party, great with patients, and just an all-around good guy. I have known physicians who were addicted to drugs, nurses who committed suicide, and respiratory therapists who smoked. This is on the same level. How do you know so much about the risks and still allow yourself to become oblivious to them?

The patient came in and was discovered to have been propelled fifteen feet from the bike. He was extremely fortunate not to have had his groin snagged by the handlebars on the way by. He ended up with a broken neck and several broken bones in his arms and legs. He had not been wearing a helmet. He was temporarily paralyzed and required a four-month hospitalization with massive rehabilitation. He has regained sufficient function to care for himself, but he will live the remainder of his life in pain.

The intersection between health and happiness is a tricky one to navigate. It's not too much to ask to want to live life on your terms, but is it too much to ask that you do so with a nod to easily learned lessons about how to do so without being reckless? Did he not realize that he wasn't just hurting himself? Did he not understand how much his co-workers and patients needed the light that emanated from him daily? This is not a cautionary tale. He was already empowered with that information. This is a tale about the consequences of our choices.

Dorsal Slit

It's the middle of the night in the emergency room; in comes a very frustrated and concerned mother. Her child has been crying uncontrollably, and she's at wit's end trying to figure out what to do. She just looks at me and asks me to help.

Babies with inconsolable crying are a common occurrence. Colic is not just crying. It's a specific type and duration of crying. However, to a concerned mother, that's irrelevant. She has a problem NOW!

There's an applicable rule of emergency medicine here: when you have a crying infant and don't have an obvious answer, check under the diaper.

There are several potential problems:

- There's the anal fissure, which is a skin tear usually caused by hard stools.
- There's the penis that can get choked, if not strangulated, by a loose hair.
- The child could have a hernia in the groin.
- The testes could be twisted.

Then there's the problem this infant had.

When examining this child, I noticed that he wasn't circumcised. That wasn't the only issue with his penis. The foreskin was engorged and trapped below the level of the glans (head of the) penis. This condition is called *paraphimosis* and is an emergency because the engorgement can cause significant cell damage (and even death; this is called *necrosis*) of the penis due to loss of the blood supply. An easy way to think about it is to consider the foreskin as choking off the head of the penis.

There are several ways to address the problem, none of which sounds good to a mother, but all of which sound better than losing one's penis.

- I tried to apply pressure to the engorged area in an effort to manually decompress the foreskin and reapply it over the entire penis. This was unsuccessful.
- I then took the smallest needle we had and created a few punctures into the engorged areas. This is done to try to release enough of the fluid so that manual decompression can be attempted again. This didn't get the job done.
- The other immediate option is called a *dorsal slit*. After appropriate precautions and preparations (include applying some local anesthesia), one quick incision along the upper portion of the foreskin relieves the pressure and the emergency. The child tolerated the procedure well.

The mother wasn't quite sure what to make of it all. She trusted that an emergency existed. She was able to see it with her own two eyes. On the other hand, her child's foreskin had just been sliced. Then she noticed that despite being cut, the child had actually stopped crying. All's well that ends well. Now, they both could get some sleep.

He Drank Himself Blind

—⋀⋁⋀—

Sometimes, when you see hysterical patients, you would do well to appreciate that some stories are so over-the-top that they just could be true.

A disheveled man comes in via ambulance yelling and out of control, saying that he can't see. The paramedics shrug at me, saying that he smells of alcohol. Sometimes patients' concerns are disregarded because of their state of intoxication—this is often a mistake. We rush him into a room and get him undressed.

There are many causes of sudden onset of vision loss, and they are already dancing through my head. However, first things first.

> Sir, I'm Dr. Sterling. I can't help you until you calm down. What happened to you?

> I can't see. I don't know what happened.

> His speech is slurred. The possibility of a stroke is real, but he doesn't have any facial droop or extremity weakness . . .

> Sir, how much alcohol have you had to drink?

> I haven't had any booze.

That was the wrong question. It doesn't take alcohol to make you "drunk." There is a class of substances known as *toxic alcohols*. (No, this doesn't have anything to do with the brand or amount of liquor consumed. The alcohol we drink socially is ethanol.) Methanol is the most dangerous of the toxic alcohols because of the substances into which it's metabolized. Methanol is contained within substances such as paint thinner, gasoline additives, wood alcohol, and window washer solvent. Yes, there are people so hard off that they will drink these substances, and yes, drinking these substances can have devastating consequences.

As it turns out, this gentleman had been on a bit of a bender and had been ingesting window washer solvent for the last day or two. This fits the story nicely because the visual complications of methanol poisoning take approximately twelve to eighteen hours to take hold. Actually, his symptoms weren't as bad as they could have been, because he had also been drinking alcohol—*huh?* I will come to that momentarily.

Currently, there exists an antidote for methanol poisoning. Back in the early days of my career, emergency room treatment of severe methanol poisoning involved receiving emergency dialysis or, if dialysis wasn't available, administration of alcohol. As many of you know, dialysis is a process by which poisons and other unwanted substances can be directly removed from the bloodstream. If dialysis is available, it's a valuable treatment tool.

The alcohol option works differently. Once alcohol (that is, ethanol) enters your bloodstream, it actually competes with toxic alcohols such as methanol for the enzyme necessary to break methanol down into its toxic byproducts. The enzyme actually prefers ethanol instead of methanol (who doesn't?), so whenever alcohol is present, methanol will end up largely being eliminated without causing much damage. Thus, a key to successful treatment is getting ethanol on board before too much methanol has been absorbed and metabolized.

Another really interesting aspect of treating these patients with the alcohol option is that it occurs in one of two ways. One prefers to give a medically precise ethanol solution, administered via IV fluids. Unfortunately, depending on the hospital (or the number of alcoholics present in the midst of either alcohol withdrawal or the effects of a toxic alcohol), the solution, which is famously known in emergency rooms as *D5E5* (5 percent dextrose and 5 percent ethanol; dextrose is a common sugar), may not be available. So what option is left? You guessed it. Send a staff member (over age twenty-one, of course) across the street to get the most potent alcohol available. Taste wasn't a consideration; it was going to be administered directly into the stomach via a tube inserted through the nose.

As interesting as the case was, it didn't have the best out-come. Treatment of alcohol poisoning occurs best when done immediately. Waiting until inflammation of the pancreas, visual difficulties, or any of the other dangerous symptoms of toxic alcohol ingestion show up is not going to end well in most cases. Of course, with many alcoholics, drinking and then blacking out is a common occurrence, and this happenstance robs patients of valuable time that, if they were being treated instead, would give them a better chance of recovery. This patient lived but had permanent visual damage.

Spousal Abuse—When Enough Is Enough

Domestic violence is in the news every day, it seems. Even so, the complexities of any individual story rarely get told. Domestic violence includes physical acts, the wounds of which are visible and dramatic. However, the mental components of abuse are often as powerful to the patient affected.

You know the story. There's a family. There's a dominating and controlling partner. There's an abusive partner. There's a submissive partner. There are physical and/or mental threats and assaults. There are feelings of hopelessness and helplessness.

There are clear risks: drugs and alcohol can exacerbate an already volatile situation. Pregnancy is a particularly sensitive time; during pregnancy, emotions are heightened, and abuse may start, increase, or intensify. Those with fewer resources or greater perceived vulnerability, such as those with physical or psychiatric disabilities or those living below the poverty line, are at even greater risk for domestic violence and lifetime risk.

It is estimated that approximately 25 percent of women who present to emergency rooms are or have been victims of domestic violence. It is an insidious condition that often goes unrevealed or is underreported, and in an overwhelming percentage of cases, evidence isn't sufficient to gain a conviction. Now, men suffer from domestic violence as well, but not with the same frequency as women and more often in a different way, which brings up the need to appreciate the range of activities inherent in the term *violence*. Women are often abused, and their suffering is typically hidden. The emergency department teams often uncover cases that otherwise would have gone unreported. In my career, the cases of domestic violence against men were of a different quality.

I have seen multiple men who were simultaneously perpetrators and subsequent victims of domestic violence. The cases involved stabbings, shootings, blunt trauma to the head (including a skillet and a baseball bat), and burns. It seems that in many cases, at some point, the abusive components of domestic violence are going to escalate. Unfortunately, this often results in the death of the individuals being abused (often at the time of trying to escape the situation), but there are many examples of when the victim has had enough and goes on the offensive or simply does what is deemed necessary to protect him- or herself. In these instances, it is psychologically understandable that the release of all that pent-up fear, frustration, and anger can have devastating consequences.

This certainly is not to suggest that one form of domestic violence is more or less forgivable or understandable. As physicians, when a patient is presenting to the emergency room dying from a bleed within the skull from blunt trauma, it's not our job to judge; it's time to treat, as a life often is in the balance. So, to those of you who are victims or perpetrators of domestic violence, be advised. Seek help before it's too late. The consequences are real, and they're real dangerous.

Choosing How You Die

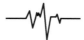

It's 6:00 a.m. in the morning. No one ever comes into the ER at 6:00 a.m. in the morning for any good reason. I get pulled out of my slumber because of a dialysis patient (due to end-stage kidney disease) coming in by ambulance because he has had a cardiac arrest. His heart has stopped functioning normally, and he's not breathing on his own. He had just been placed into a nursing home about five days ago.

When he arrives to the emergency room, there's the typical controlled chaos. The paramedics haven't been able to intubate him, nor have they been able to put in an IV, which is needed to give blood and medicine. The cardiac monitor shows a rhythm that looks like a malignant *arrhythmia*, which is an abnormal heart rate that eventually leads to the heart stopping.

It looks like there's work to be done.

In pretty short order (meaning within a minute or two):

- We get the patient intubated (we place a breathing tube down his throat to maintain delivery of oxygen to his lungs and throughout his body).
- We place a central IV line (a special tube with a shorter route to the heart).

Now, about that heart rhythm . . .

I already know this isn't a typical cardiac arrest in progress. The applicable rule of emergency medicine here is that cardiac arrests in dialysis patients are typically due to abnormally high potassium levels until proven otherwise. Patients with high potassium levels display a variety of abnormal heart rhythms, culminating in a rhythm that's nearly identical to the rhythm seen in certain patients in cardiac arrest. These two types of patients have completely different treatment needs, so it's important to understand this.

In pretty short order, the patient receives a series of medicines that reverse and lower the high potassium levels, returning him to a normal heart rhythm, and he proceeds to normalize.

This patient didn't present to the emergency room on accident. As mentioned, this relatively young man had been placed in a nursing home approximately five days before this episode due to frustration over the status of his kidneys and increasing noncompliance with his treatment regimen. In fact, he had refused to receive his last few rounds of dialysis. The purpose of dialysis is to eliminate waste from the body due to the kidney's inability to do so; if the kidneys aren't working and you're not getting dialysis, this is what happens next.

In talking with his family, it was evident that this patient was passive-aggressively exercising his wish to end his life. His depression had slowly progressed since being placed on dialysis, to where his presentation must have been an intentional cry for death.

Many patients choose how they are going to die well in advance of the time of death. As a society and within our families, we (perhaps subconsciously) don't allow these conversations to be held. It's as if we don't trust ourselves and the decisions we have made about how we live our lives, as well as how that translates into how we will die. It's also as if we still trust the magic of medicine to pull us out of whatever hole we have spent our lives digging for ourselves.

It's not just patients who commit suicide abruptly that have made a choice. In this day and age, smokers have to be aware that they are likely going to die from lung cancer or emphysema, strokes, or a heart attack. The morbidly obese by choice have made certain decisions about how they are going to die. These situations play out all day every day in the emergency room. It seems like we should allow for a difference between a patient with a mental illness whose effort to end his or her life is due to chemical imbalances in the brain and a person living out a lifestyle based on choices.

Isn't it interesting that when the time comes, we will humanely take a wounded or dying pet animal out of its misery, but we won't offer the same accommodation for humans?

The Greatest Miracle

I have only two or three health-related fears. I know I have pre-pared myself to handle whatever comes in a way that I will have the best chance possible of surviving anything short of getting eaten by a shark or something crazy like that. It's the things you can't control that give you pause. The line in the serenity prayer about having the serenity to accept things you can't control is a very heavy lift when you're up against it. I have stared in the face what was once my greatest fear: my mother's death.

My mother has a combination of medical conditions, in-cluding congestive heart failure and atrial fibrillation. The total of these conditions renders her heart less than normally able to pump strongly. In fact, it sometimes has the type of quivering motion and suboptimal blood flow that leads to blood clots. To combat this, she and other patients like her are often placed on blood thinners. When you're eighty years old, this is a setup for problems that can come from several directions.

I'm a thousand miles away, and I get a phone call that she's in an emergency room. She apparently had an episode of massive bleeding from her stomach caused by the blood thinner. The loss of blood caused her to fall to the ground. She may or may not have hit her head, but either way, she ended up with a massive bleed inside the brain known as a *subdural hematoma*. The amount of blood inside of her brain took up so much space that it shifted the contents of the brain out of place (this is what's known as *herniation*) enough to cause a coma. To place this in proper perspective, a subdural hematoma comes with a mortality (death) rate of 80 percent by itself. When it occurs in an eighty-year-old with herniation, atrial fibrillation, congestive heart failure, and the other complications, the death rate is 99.9 percent (it had previously been 100 percent).

I was in a location where it took me about eight hours to get back to Chicago. That gave me enough time to collect myself and my thoughts. I was going home to bury my mother. There was no uncertainty in my mind about this. It was the single most miserable feeling of my life. However, that was very selfish of me. I have long thought that my mother was the one person I knew who was most ready to go to heaven. As long as she was at peace, I wouldn't really have a problem with letting her go.

By the time I landed, she had already had a *craniotomy*, a procedure necessary in intracranial bleeds with herniation in which holes are drilled into the brain in order to release the pressure and blood buildup. The hope is that this release of pressure will reverse the herniation and place the brain back in a normal position. The neurosurgeon and I had a prolonged conversation about the procedure. My mother's heart likely wasn't strong enough to undergo any type of surgery. The surgery itself had significant risks, and she could have died on the operating table. Even with survival, the question of quality of life is significant. How would I want her to spend her last days, knowing the amount of brain damage she had endured? How could I expect her to ever return to a normal life with the level of heart disease she already had? What were her wishes?

Everything that I knew as a physician told me that the confluence of conditions could not be survived. I knew this when I first got the call. I knew this when I saw the CT scan of her brain, shifted and misconfigured. I knew this when I saw her after surgery. I knew this even as she lay comatose for months and sustained a hospital stay for over half a year. I hadn't conceptualized that *she had survived this* until she actually left the hospital and went to a rehabilitation center. Now, several years later, she has returned to virtually the exact same person I had last seen before the accident, with no difference in memory, mental capacity, or even ability to walk. I guess I didn't know anything, and I couldn't be happier to have been so wrong!

I would like to think that any good will I have earned in twenty years of caring for others was returned, paid in full. What's more likely is that the good will my mother displayed throughout her life paid for any favors she received. Further, the healthy life lived by my mother came through for her in her time of need.

What I received was an affirmation of the same mentality I had always been willing to apply to the care of my own patients: always give patients the best possible opportunity to get through their health challenges, and things will take care of themselves. Never know so much that you deny a patient a chance for a miracle; they really do happen, despite all medical logic and knowledge to the contrary.

I can check one fear off my list. What a joy it is to have borrowed time.

About The Author

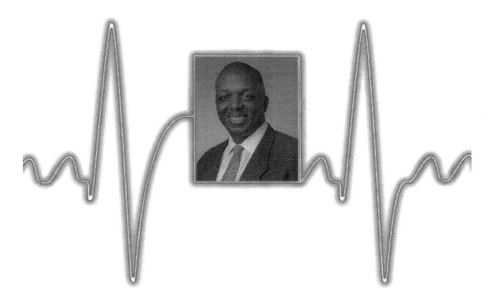

Dr. Jeffrey Sterling is a national leader in community-based medicine and health care. He serves as president and CEO of SterlingMedicalAdvice.com, a national public health initiative providing personal and immediate healthcare information and advice to consumers. Dr. Sterling also is president and CEO of Sterling Initiatives (SI), a healthcare consulting and implementation firm assisting entities with clinical, operational, and financial best practices. SI has assisted health systems, health plans, state governments, and medical practices in three dozen states and countries. SI has gained particular notoriety for its work in creating "centers of excellence" among hospitals and other healthcare entities. Dr. Sterling is also author of the healthcare blog "Straight, No Chaser" at www.jeffreysterlingmd.com.

Additionally,

- Dr. Sterling serves as president of the Northwestern University Black Alumni Association, representing over 4,500 alumni nationally organized in twenty-six local chapters.
- Dr. Sterling has served as CEO, senior VP, corporate medical officer, national physician practice director, and regional medical director for various healthcare contract management groups, and as medical director for seventeen emergency medical system units and home health companies.
- Dr. Sterling has served as chairman and/or medical director of the departments of emergency medicine at the following level I trauma emergency departments:
    - John Peter Smith Health Network (JPS) in Fort Worth, TX
    - Prince George's Hospital Center, Cheverly, MD (Metro DC)
    - St. Joseph Regional Medical Center, Milwaukee, WI.
- Dr. Sterling founded DFW Urgent Care, a series of award-winning urgent care centers in Texas, New York, and California providing quality equivalent, cost-effective care alternatives to hospital emergency rooms.
- Dr. Sterling founded the Minority Association of Pre-Health Students (MAPS), a national organization of premedical and other health career aspirants with chapters in over 300 colleges nationally.
- Dr. Sterling served as the founding medical director for JPS Health Network's Sexual Assault Nurse Examiner (SANE) program and created the first SANE program in the state of Connecticut at Connecticut Children's Medical Center.
- Dr. Sterling founded DS Comprehensive Psychological Consulting, a contract management firm providing optimization of care for those in need of acute behavioral intervention, working throughout New Mexico and Texas.

- Dr. Sterling founded US Asthma Care, a series of outcomes-based, best-practice disease management treatment facilities in Texas and Illinois working with health plans to reduce hospitalization and improve clinical outcomes among asthmatics.
- Dr. Sterling founded and served as medical director of the Covenant Healthcare Asthma Clinics in Milwaukee, then the largest asthma education clinic in Wisconsin.
- Dr. Sterling has served on the board of the Asthma & Allergy Foundation of America, Texas Chapter, and the American Lung Association, Central States Region.
- Dr. Sterling served as chairman of the DFW Minority Business Council's Health Industry Group, a consortium of over seventy healthcare business enterprises across the Dallas-Fort Worth Metroplex.

Dr. Sterling has degrees from Northwestern University, Harvard University School of Public Health (health policy management), and the University of Illinois College of Medicine, and he completed his emergency medicine residency at Cook County Hospital in Chicago.

Dr. Sterling is a speaker in high demand on topics of asthma, pneumonia, acute coronary syndromes, healthcare economics, and healthcare disparities, having delivered over one thousand lectures nationally.

Made in the USA
Middletown, DE
13 January 2018